Diabete...

Diabetic No More

Normalize Blood Sugar, Reverse Diabetes, and Say Goodbye to Drugs and Testing Forever (How to cure diabetes with healthy living and a diabetes diet)

By: Rene Gregory

DIABETIC NO MORE

Legal notice

DIABETIC NO MORE

Table of Contents

An Overview of Diabetes

Misconceptions about Diabetes

The different types of diabetes are sometimes referred to as a "group of diseases", but not all of them are. However, they are all caused by a single symptom, which is high blood glucose levels. Diabetes is when the body has excessive glucose in the blood. This can be for one of two reasons: the body isn't producing enough insulin or the body's cells are unable to absorb the glucose produced by the body.

In the United States, diabetes is the 7th highest cause of death. It's drastically underreported when it comes to cause of death, and studies have shown that of all the diabetics who die, only around 35 to 40% of them actually have diabetes listed on their death certificate, and only 10 to 15% had diabetes listed as a secondary cause of death. Keep in mind that most diabetics also have heart disease (number 1 cause of death) or cancer (number 2 cause of death) on their death certificates, rather than the underlying diabetes. If diabetes is listed at all, it is probably 3rd or 4th.

About 120 million people in the United States are classified as either prediabetic or diabetic. About 387 million people worldwide have diabetes, and about 90% of those individuals suffer from Type 2. By 2035, it is predicted that there will be 592 million individuals with diabetes. According to the Center for Disease Control (CDC), one in three of the individuals born since 2000 will get diabetes (National Diabetes Statistics Report, 2014 released June 10, 2014).

Diabetes is also expensive: in 2012 it cost $245 billion to diagnose diabetes, $176 billion to care for those afflicted, and $69 billion in lost productivity. In 2014 the global cost was about $612 billion USD. People with diabetes have medical expense that are 2.3 times higher than those without, and diabetes doubles an individual's risk of death. This is a worldwide problem, but it is more common in some countries than others. The International Diabetes Foundation lists the top ten countries that have the highest rates of diabetes, starting with the highest rates:

1. China
2. India
3. United States of America
4. Brazil
5. Russia
6. Mexico
7. Indonesia
8. Egypt
9. Japan
10. Pakistan

Diabetes is caused by high blood glucose, which is also called high blood sugar. This is caused by two main things: First, sometimes the pancreas does not produce enough insulin, which leads to an abnormal metabolism of blood sugar. Second, sometimes the pancreas produces enough insulin, but then the body's cells are unable to respond properly. People are diagnosed with diabetes if they have high blood sugar levels for a long period of time. Signs of high blood sugar include increased thirst, increased hunger, and frequent urination. If diabetes isn't treated, it can lead to many health issues. Some of acute complications are nonketotic hyperosmolar coma, diabetic ketoacidosis coma, and death. Some other long-term complications include:

- Stroke and heart disease: Diabetes increases the risk of both by threefold.
- High blood pressure: Three-fourths of diabetics also struggle with high blood pressure, which is pressure at 130/80 or more.
- Kidney disease: Kidney failure is often caused by diabetes.
- Nervous system damage: Most diabetics suffer from nervous system damage, such as erectile dysfunction disorder, reduced feeling in the feet, and impaired digestion.
- Foot ulcers and amputation: Diabetes is the main cause for limb amputations.
- Eye damage: Most adults who lose their eyesight can blame diabetes.
- Cancer: Individuals with diabetes are at an increased risk for cancer. It increases the risk of bladder, colorectal, and breast cancer by 20 to 50%. It doubles the risk of endometrial, pancreatic, and liver cancer.

There are also a few different types of diabetes. Prediabetes is when an individual's blood glucose levels are higher than they should be, but not high enough to be diagnosed with Type 2 diabetes. With lifestyle changes, an individual can prevent and reverse this diagnosis.

Type 2 diabetes is when an individual's blood glucose levels are high enough for long enough that it is dangerous. At this point, medical treatment is required. Type 2 diabetes is the most common, and with 90% of all diabetics diagnosed with Type 2 worldwide, it has reached epidemic proportions. With lifestyle changes, an individual can prevent and reverse this diagnosis.

Type 1 diabetes occurs when the pancreas produces insulin, which produces beta cells, but an autoimmune reaction destroys the insulin. This can have one of two effects: either the pancreas can't keep up and produce enough insulin to carry blood glucose to the body's cells, or it stops producing insulin altogether. Type 1 can also be caused by the body's cells being unable to respond to the insulin properly. In Europe and North America, 5% of all diabetics suffer from Type 1. If Type 1 sufferers are still able to produce some insulin, they may be able to implement lifestyle changes and regenerate their pancreas to the point where they have normal blood sugar levels.

Latent Autoimmune Diabetes of Adults (LADA) occurs when adults develop Type 1 diabetes. Adults with LADA are sometimes mistakenly diagnosed with Type 2. This occurs because their age is noticed more than their symptoms. LADA sufferers might be able to achieve regular blood sugar levels with serious lifestyle changes.

When a pregnant woman without any previous history of diabetes develops high blood sugar, it is called gestational diabetes. Gestational diabetes is similar to Type 2 because it occurs due to cellular responsiveness issues and inadequate insulin production. It occurs in around 10% of pregnancies, and it generally goes away after the baby is born. However, about 5 to 10% of women who get gestational diabetes then develop diabetes, generally Type 2. Gestational diabetes can be treated with lifestyle changes, but it also requires medical supervision throughout the pregnancy.

Untreated diabetes often comes with the following symptoms: weight loss, stupor, lethargy, polyphagia (increased hunger), polydipsia (increased thirst), an acetone smell on the breath, Kussmaul breathing, which is labored and deep breathing, and polyuria, which is frequent urination and the body's attempts to expel the extra glucose by drawing water from the cells to the bloodstream. There are several other symptoms that can hint towards diabetes, but they are not exclusive to this condition. More symptoms include headaches, slow-healing cuts, nausea, vomiting, itchy skin, chronic fatigue, abdominal pain, and blurry vision that can reach blindness.

Type 1 diabetes occurs suddenly, generally in children who are average or underweight. Ketoacidosis is common, autoantibodies are usually present, and endogenous insulin is either low or nonexistent. Also, the concordance in identical twins is 50% and the prevalence is around 10%. Type 2 diabetes sets in gradually, generally in adults who are overweight. Ketoacidosis is rare, autoantibodies are absent, and endogenous insulin can be normal, increased, or decreased. Also, the concordance in identical twins is 90% and the prevalence is around 90% as well. The following tests can be used to diagnose diabetes:

1. The Fasting Plasma Glucose (FPG) test measures an individual's blood sugar after they have fasted. If the fasting blood sugar

level is between 100 and 125 mg/dl, prediabetes is diagnosed. If it measures more than 126 mg/dl, it is diabetes.

2. Oral glucose tolerance testing (OGTT) takes around 2 hours, and it doesn't have a prognostic to measure an individual's insulin response to high glucose levels. During an OGTT test, individuals are given glucose so that doctors can measure their blood glucose level. If the glucose level rises to around 140 ml/dl, it is prediabetes. If the glucose level rises to 199 ml/dl and stays there, it is diabetes. Diabetes is also diagnosed if the levels reaches 200 mg/dl or higher.

3. Glycated Hemoglobin (HbAlc) test is used to diagnose less severe cases of diabetes. Doctors use this test to estimate your average blood glucose level for the last few months. Generally around 4 to 6% of hemoglobin is glycosylated, which means that the average blood glucose level is between 60 and 120 mg/dl. HbA1c is increased to 8 or 10% with mild hyperglycemia, and severe hyperglycemia can get it up to 20%. Diabetics should try to keep their HbA1c levels to 7% or less, which is a blood glucose level of no more than 150 mg/dl.

Blood sugar levels need to be confirmed on a different day using one of the above before diabetes is diagnosed. It is best and easiest to measure an individual who is fasting at 126mg/dl above plasma glucose levels.

Prediabetes

Prediabetes is mainly caused by lack of exercise, excess carbohydrate consumption, and obesity. It is when the fasting blood sugar level is higher than normal, but it's not high enough to be considered diabetes (which is in the 101 mg/dl to 125 mg/dl range). Prediabetes is a difficult condition to diagnose, as it has no symptoms besides some abnormal carbohydrate digestion. Generally speaking, you can expect Type 2 diabetes to develop after prediabetes, but some people stay in the prediabetes state for years before signs of Type 2 diabetes start to show.

Most people who have prediabetes are unaware of it and undiagnosed. However, if you test yourself (you can find these online) or go to a doctor and discover prediabetes, it is easy to reverse your blood sugar levels and prevent the onset of Type 2 diabetes by implementing some lifestyle changes. These include losing some weight, exercising more, and eating a diabetes-friendly diet.

In the United States, about 86 million individuals over 20 years old have prediabetes. Reversing this diagnosis helps avoid serious health problems down the road, such as Type 2 diabetes and issues with eyes, limbs, blood vessels, heart, and kidneys. By the time diabetes had been diagnosed, many of these life-threatening issues have already gained a foothold.

The following are some factors that make you more likely to develop prediabetes:

- You are woman who had gestational diabetes or gave birth to a baby weighing over 9 pounds.
- You are a woman with Polycystic Ovary Syndrome (PCOS).
- You are Native American, African-American, Hispanic, Pacific Islander, or Asian American.
- You have low HDL cholesterol, high triglycerides, high LDL cholesterol, or cholesterol over 300.
- You have a family history of Type 2 diabetes.
- You are obese or overweight, especially around the belly area. For some people, even a small amount of weight gain can lead to prediabetes or progression to Type 2 diabetes.
- You are 45 years old or older.
- You don't exercise.
- Your diet is high in carbohydrates.

Even just five pounds of excess body fat can make it difficult for insulin to bring glucose to the body's cells. Excess body fat interferes in multiple ways, and insulin also has a harder time doing its job when an individual overeats, eats fatty foods, or eats low-nutrient foods.

NOTE: However, you shouldn't give overweight diabetic people insulin, as it makes them more diabetic, promotes weight gain, and ultimately makes them sicker. This piece is intended to help prediabetic and diabetic patients understand their condition and make good choices about their blood sugar levels in order to help control their diabetes.

If you meet any of these criteria and also have heart disease, signs of insulin resistance, and a history of abnormal blood sugar, you should be tested for prediabetes.

Insulin resistance is when your body produces insulin, but then doesn't respond the way it should. Generally, individuals with prediabetes don't have symptoms, but blurred vision, chronic fatigue, increased urination, or increased thirst can all be indicators. You or your doctor can use three different tests to determine if prediabetes is a concern:

1. Fasting Plasma Glucose Test: This test has you fast for 8 hours, then it measures your blood sugar. If it is higher than normal but not high enough to be diabetes (below 101 mg/dl and 125 mg/dl), you might have prediabetes.
2. Oral Glucose Tolerance Test: This test has you fast of 8 hours, then it tests your blood sugar. Then you have a sweet drink, fast for another 2 hours, and test your blood sugar again. If your blood sugar is higher than normal after the 2 hours, you might have prediabetes.
3. Glycated Hemoglobin (HbA1c) Test: This test has you look at your average blood sugar over the past two or three months. You can use it to diagnose diabetes or determine whether or not your diabetes is under control.
4. Blood Sugar Self-Testing lets you test yourself at home if you want to avoid the expenses and having a medical record of diabetes testing.

Prediabetes isn't treated with medicine, instead it is treated with lifestyle changes. These include:

- Losing weight (losing 5 to 10% of your weight can make a huge different).

- Eating a healthy, low carb, high protein, quality fat, diabetic diet.
- Stop smoking.
- Exercising (find something that you like so that you will do it every day without finding excuses or worrying about weather - dancing, lifting weights, rebounding).
- Get enough sleep.
- Treat hypertension (high blood pressure) and high cholesterol by getting off statin and hypertension drugs.
- Reduce stress in your life

Type 2 Diabetes

Type 2 diabetes is when the pancreas stops producing insulin or the body becomes resistant to insulin. Either way, the body's cells are not receiving glucose from insulin, which means that the sugar levels in your blood increase. As this happens, the beta cells in the pancreas produce more insulin, but eventually they become impaired and can't keep up with the body's demand for it.

If an individual fasts and then tests show a blood sugar level higher than prediabetic levels (more than 125 mg/dl), they have Type 2 diabetes. Type 2 diabetes used to be known as adult-onset diabetes or non-insulin-dependent diabetes mellitus (NIDDM). It has had a dramatic increase in diagnoses in the past five years. It's more common for people age 45 and up, but more and more children are being diagnosed with it as well.

Treatment options include medications (pills), lifestyle changes (losing weight, quitting smoking, exercising, changing your diet, getting enough sleep), and possibly insulin injections. Many doctors are misinformed and go straight for medication options, but you need to find a doctor who wants to try lifestyle changes first, as that's the better option.

Taking pills can lead to a dependence on medication, negative long term consequences, and issues with side effects. Lifestyle changes don't come with these concerns, so it's the preferable option. Medication and insulin can sometimes actually make things worse by increasing your blood sugar, along with other side effects.

As glucose builds in your blood instead of being taken in by cells, it can starve your cells of energy and make you feel fatigued. If you have high blood glucose levels for too long, it can hurt your body and have a negative impact on your kidneys, eyes, heart, and nerves - it can even lead to death. Generally, Type 2 gets worse over time. However, with treatment options, it is possible to keep your blood sugar at normal levels. Many people are able to stay healthy just by sticking to a specific diet and exercising.

Researchers aren't entirely sure what causes Type 2 diabetes to develop, but usually carbohydrate digestion is abnormal, along with other symptoms. However, they do know what factors put people at a greater risk for diabetes. Let's take a look at some of them:

- Weight: Being overweight or obese is the main factor that puts people at risk for developing Type 2 diabetes. As your body gains fatty tissue, your cells become more resistant to insulin. However, an individual does not have to be overweight to get diabetes.
- Stress: Both mental and physical stress are risky.
- Smoking: Smoking is a very risky activity. Cigarettes contains nicotine, which hardens and narrows your blood vessels. This makes is more difficult for your body to pump blood, which will only add to the increased risk of heart disease that comes with diabetes.
- Lack of exercise: The less active your lifestyle is, the greater your risk for developing Type 2 diabetes. Exercise is important for helping you control your weight, making your cells more sensitive to insulin, and using your blood glucose for energy.
- Family history: If one of your parents or siblings has diabetes, you are more likely to get it.
- Lack of sleep: Getting enough quality sleep is important for making sure that your body functions properly.
- Fat distribution: If most of your fat is stored in your abdomen rather than your thighs or hips, you are at a greater risk for Type 2 diabetes.
- Age: After age 45 people are more susceptible to Type 2 diabetes. As people age, they lose muscle mass, exercise less, and gain weight. However, diagnoses in younger people and even children are becoming more common.

- Race: We're not quite sure why individuals of different races are more likely to develop diabetes, but Pacific Islanders, Hispanics, American Indians, Blacks, and Asian Americans are all more likely to get diabetes.
- Diet: The following are all associated with diabetes: rice, white flour, potatoes, bread, pasta, and other complex carbohydrates, sugary processed foods, fig-sweetened drinks, trans fats, saturated fats, salad dressings, fatty fried foods, vegetable oil, corn oil, soybean oil, and cottonseed oil. For an alternative to the oils, try extra virgin olive oil or coconut oil.
- Gestational diabetes: If a woman has gestational diabetes when she is pregnant, she is more likely to develop Type 2 diabetes. If a woman has a baby who is more than 9 pounds, she is more likely to develop Type 2 diabetes.
- Prediabetes: Individuals with prediabetes have blood sugar levels that are higher than normal, but not to the point of a diabetes diagnosis. If you don't take steps to handle prediabetes, it will probably progress to Type 2 diabetes.
- High blood pressure medications: These are medications for hypertension, and diabetes is very closely associated with heart disease.
- High cholesterol medications: These are also called statins, and they are known to cause diabetes.
- Polycystic ovary syndrome: This is a condition that makes women have excess hair growth, irregular menstrual periods, and obesity issues, and it also increases their risk for diabetes.

Individuals with Type 2 diabetes should avoid therapies and drugs that increase insulin levels, as Type 2 is characterized by high insulin and glucose levels. Type 2 treatment should focus on lifestyle changes. Strategies such as diet, weight loss, and exercise can all help increase your body's sensitivity to insulin. Type 2 diabetes generally develops slowly, and the symptoms we discussed might be difficult to spot, or not there at all. They start out very slowly, and an individual might have Type 2 diabetes for years before they become aware of it. Watch out for the following symptoms:

- Increased hunger: When there isn't enough insulin available to move sugar into the body's cells, they become depleted of energy and you eat more to make up for it.
- Hyperglycemia: This refers to increased thirst and urination. When extra sugar collects in your bloodstream, it pulls fluid from the tissues and makes you thirsty. When you drink more, you end up urinating more. Also, your body tries to dilute the high blood sugar by pulling water from the cells and urinating it out. This results in high levels of glucose in the urine, which also results in a decrease in calories.
- Blurred vision: If your blood sugar is too high, your body pulls fluid from your eye lenses to help, which can make it more difficult for you to focus.
- Chronic Fatigue: When your body's cells are deprived of the sugar they need, you can become tired and irritable.
- Weight loss: Individuals with diabetes might lose some weight because their body can't

metabolize glucose, so it turns to alternative fuels such as fat and muscle.

- Acanthosis nigricans: This is a condition where individuals start to find darker patches of velvety skin in various creases and folds, such as around the neck and in the armpits. Some people with Type 2 diabetes have this, as it indicates a resistance to insulin.
- Frequent infections or slow-healing cuts: Diabetes hurts your ability to resist infections and heal wounds.

Type 2 diabetes can be diagnosed in a few different ways, three require a doctor and one can be done at home by yourself. Type 2 can be treated without the risky drugs, but that option requires a strict nutritional plan and lifestyle changes, as well as supervision and support from a doctor. Many misinformed doctors go straight for medication, so find somebody who is open to trying lifestyle changes first.

1. Fasting Plasma Glucose Test: This test has you fast for eight hours and then measure your blood sugar. If it's higher than normal (101 mg/dl or more) and lower than a diabetes level (125 mg/dl), you have prediabetes. If you are 126 mg/dl or higher, you have Type 2 diabetes. Either way, your doctor should recommend some serious lifestyle and diet changes before they resort to drugs.
2. Oral Glucose Tolerance Test: This test has you fast for eight hours, then it records your blood sugar. Then you have a sugary drink, fast for another two hours, and test your levels again. If your blood

sugar is over 126 mg/dl after the additional two hours, you might have Type 2 diabetes.

3. Hemoglobin A1C Test: This test looks at your average blood sugar levels for the previous 2 to 3 months. It is often used to figure out whether or not an individual's diabetes is under control, but it can also be used to diagnose it.

4. Blood Sugar Self-Testing: Medical expenses can get a little difficult, and diabetes testing shows up on your medical record, so testing yourself at home is always a possibility.

Type 1 Diabetes

When individuals have Type 1 diabetes, their immune system has turned against itself and started destroying the body's cells. This is called an autoimmune disease, and with Type 1 it means that cells found in the pancreas called beta cells, or b cells, are destroyed. Beta cells are responsible for producing insulin, and insulin delivers glucose to body cells. This type of diabetes used to be known as Insulin Dependent Diabetes Mellitus (IDDM) or Juvenile Diabetes, since most cases occurred in children.

Around 10% of all diabetics have Type 1 diabetes. It's more common in individuals who are of northern European descent, and less common in individuals of Asian or Middle Eastern descent. Most Type 1 diabetics have a healthy weight and a healthy body when the disease starts to take control. Type 1 diabetes is not caused by obesity, but is dangerous for anybody with the disease to be overweight.

In the early stages of treatment, responsiveness and sensitivity to insulin are usually normal. Symptoms may take weeks or months to become severe. The traditional treatment for Type 1 diabetes includes medication in the form of pills, insulin in the form of injections, and lifestyle changes such as changes in exercise levels, diet, smoking, weight, and sleep. Keep in mind, however, that medications and insulin have side effects, and sometime they can even lead to reverse effects and low blood sugar.

If Type 1 diabetes is mild and the pancreas is still producing some insulin, individuals may be able to regain normal blood sugar levels by using micronutrients to fortify their immune systems. This gives the pancreas a chance to slow down and recover before it stops producing insulin altogether. In order to coax the pancreas into normal insulin production again, an individual must implement lifestyle changes rather than relying on therapies, drugs, and insulin.

Most Type 1 diabetics need to take at least some insulin because their pancreas has stopped producing it completely. However, if they stick to a diabetic diet, they can reduce the amount of insulin needed. A diabetic diet can also help prevent even more serious health issues later on. A third of Type 1 diabetics die before they reach 50 years old, but changing to a healthier lifestyle can help prevent this, and one of these changes includes a change in diet. A nutritious diabetic diet can reduce the need for insulin, and it helps to prevent drastic and dangerous changes in blood glucose levels.

Type 1 diabetes can be caused by genetics, exposure to certain immunizations and viruses, and many other factors. It generally occurs during childhood or adolescence, but some adults get it as well. The symptoms can appear quickly and can include: increased thirst, hunger, and urination, unintended weight loss, weakness and fatigue, vaginal yeast infections, blurred vision, mood changes, and new instances of bedwetting. If you notice any of these signs in your child or yourself, visit your doctor. There are a few different tests that can be performed to diagnose Type 1 diabetes.

1. Fasting Plasma Glucose Test: This test has you fast for eight hours, then it measures your blood sugar.
2. Oral Glucose Tolerance Test: This test has you fast for eight hours, then it measures your blood sugar. Next you have a very sweet drink and fast for another two hours, then measure your blood sugar levels again.
3. Hemoglobin A1C Test: This test looks at your average blood sugar levels for the past two or three months. It can be used to diagnose diabetes, but it can also be used to find out whether your diabetes is under control.
4. Blood Sugar testing at Home: If you don't want to pay medical expenses or have diabetes listed on your medical records, you can test yourself at home.

It might be possible to treat Type 1 with minimal amounts of insulin and medications. You can avoid both if your pancreas is still producing some insulin, but you still need to monitor your blood sugar levels carefully and maintain a very strict diet and lifestyle. Lifestyle and nutrition changes are a better idea than using insulin, yet many misinformed doctors will suggest medications right away. If your doctor directs you to medication first, you will need to find a new doctor. If a person with Type 1 diabetes also has severe complications, some undergo a pancreas transplant. It can also lead to end stage kidney disease, which requires a kidney transplant.

Many people with Type 1 diabetes say that having the condition is like having another job, and it's true that administering insulin and monitoring your blood sugar levels can be very stressful. New inventions such as the Bionic Pancreas may help to ease the burdens of diabetes. The Bionic Pancreas is a device which is able to mimic a real pancreas. It delivers insulin to maintain lower blood sugar levels, and glucagon to raise them if needed. You can find out more about this invention online.

Latent Autoimmune Diabetes of Adults (LADA)

LADA is simply Type 1 diabetes, but it is diagnosed in adults instead of children. LADA is often misdiagnosed as Type 2 diabetes, since adults are far less likely to get the disease. Individuals with mild cases of LADA are still able to produce insulin in their pancreas, and they might be able to reach normal blood sugar levels again. However, they need to avoid using therapies, drugs, or injections to increase their insulin. Instead, they must focus on strict and aggressive lifestyle and nutrition changes if they want their pancreas to be able to function normally again. LADA might be treatable without drugs or insulin at this point, but again, only if their pancreas is still producing some insulin, and individuals will require close medical supervision through everything.

Keep in mind that this only possible with mild cases, and most LADA diabetics will require insulin injections for the rest of their lives - these are the individuals who can no longer produce any insulin. Lifestyle and nutrition changes are preferable to insulin and medication, but many misinformed doctors go straight for drugs. If your doctor wants to start with medications rather than lifestyle changes, find a new one. Some LASA patients who also have severe complications need a pancreas transplant, and a kidney transplant may be required for people who reach the point of end stage kidney disease.

Many people with LADA say that having the condition is like having another job, and it's true that administering insulin and monitoring your blood sugar levels can be very stressful. New inventions such as the Bionic Pancreas may help to ease the burdens of diabetes. The Bionic Pancreas is a device which is able to mimic a real pancreas. It delivers insulin to maintain lower blood sugar levels, and glucagon to raise them if needed. You can find out more about this invention online.

Gestational Diabetes

When a pregnant woman, with no prior diabetic history, develops blood sugar levels that are in the diabetic range, this is considered gestational diabetes. With the combination of both a comparably deficient secretion of insulin as well as how the insulin reacts within the body, gestational diabetes highly resembles Type 2 diabetes. As many as 10% of all pregnancies result in gestational diabetes with most conditions resolving after the baby is born. However, even after the birthing process, about 5-10% of women who developed gestational diabetes wind up obtaining another form of diabetes, more often than not it will be Type 2. Women who are overweight have a greater risk factor in developing gestational diabetes, though, for any women who are diagnosed with diabetes during their pregnancy, this can be a risk factor for their future pregnancies as well as increase their probability of developing a type of diabetes later in their lifetime. The elevations of glucose throughout pregnancy increases overall birth weight, causing possible complications that lead to the need for a C-section delivery. The possibility of having high blood pressure, as well as having an excessive amount of amniotic fluid surrounding the baby, is increased by this higher glucose level. The baby can also suffer from higher risks of central nervous system abnormalities, malformations of the skeletal muscles and congenital heart disease. The increase of fetal insulin may also cause respiratory distress syndrome. High blood bilirubin levels can occur from excessive red blood cell destruction, as bilirubin is a pigmentation that is normally made from the breakdown of these blood cells. Perinatal death (considered five months before birth or one month after) can occur in severe cases. The children who are born to mothers who had gestational diabetes during their pregnancy have a greater risk of developing diabetes themselves, as well as an increased risk of obesity. These same children also have a higher risk of obtaining neonatal jaundice and hypoglycemia.

Diagnosing Gestational Diabetes

There are three different blood test that your doctor can perform to check for gestational diabetes. There are also means by which you can test yourself at home. The Fasting Plasma Glucose Test measures blood sugar levels after fasting for eight hours. If levels are higher than normal rates (70-100 mg/dL) but below diabetic diagnosis levels (>125 mg/dL), it is possible that you may have prediabetes. The Oral Glucose Tolerance Test records blood sugar after fasting for eight hours and then, again, two hours after having a very sweet drink. If blood sugar readings are greater than normal after the two hours following the test, this could also be an indicator of prediabetes. The Hemoglobin A1C Test takes a look at your blood sugar averages for the prior two to three months. This can be utilized to diagnose diabetes or even see if a preexisting condition is being properly controlled. There are many different websites that people can use from home to test themselves for the possibility of having diabetes. Most do this in order to cut costs on medical expenses or to avoid the result showing up on their medical records.

Gestational diabetes is a condition that is treatable, but it is one that should be carefully monitored and should have comprehensive medical supervision. The traditional use of drugs to manage diabetes is an approach that is both risky and deficient. What is needed is a vigorous nutritional guide that can reverse the effects of gestational diabetes without the use of drugs that can pose risk to you and your baby. While this is a preferable means to resolve this condition, as opposed to insulin and medications, a number of doctors tend to prescribe drugs right away. If your doctor prescribes drugs without first addressing lifestyle changes and nutrition, it is advised to find a different doctor who will be more in tune to your needs.

Screening for Diabetes

There are millions of Americans, and even more around the world, who go throughout their daily lives without knowing that they have undiagnosed prediabetes or diabetes. Guidelines for the determination of who should be tested is crucial. Body Mass Index, or BMI, measures one's weight in relation to their height. This is an aid in determining whether people, ages 20 and older, are underweight, of normal weight, overweight, or deemed obese. You can calculate your own BMI by clicking on the following link and comparing your BMI rating to the weight ranges listed: http://www.whathealth.com/bmi/calculator.html.

Once your BMI number rating is determined, compare it to these weight statuses to determine which category you fall into: Underweight - BMI calculation below 18.5, Normal Weight - BMI calculation between 18.5 and 24.9, Overweight - BMI calculation between 25 and 29.9, Obese - BMI calculation of 30 or greater. A disadvantage of BMI calculation is that it can overestimate overall body fat in athletic or muscular individuals, categorizing them as overweight. In fact, bodybuilders are often wrongfully categorized within the obese range. Another issue with BMI calculation is that it can also underestimate overall body fat in those who have muscle wasting, which often occurs with the elderly.

Diabetic and prediabetic screenings should be conducted for adults of any age that have a BMI greater or equal to 25 and who have one, or more, of the following risk factors: physical inactivity, a high risk race (Asian American, African American, Native American, Pacific Islander or Latino), a first-degree relative with diabetes (father, mother or sibling), a mother who previously gave birth to a baby that weighed more than nine pounds or who had been diagnosed previously with gestational diabetes, polycystic ovarian syndrome, A1C blood glucose levels greater than 5.7, a total cholesterol that is greater than 200, hypertension or anyone on hypertensive medications, obesity and a history of heart disease. Another major factor for diabetes is age. Everyone, beginning at the age of 45, should be screened for diabetes even if they do not have any of the aforementioned risk factors.

How often screening will be conducted will be based on an initial screening. If the first is considered normal, your doctor should repeat testing at least every three years. If there are a multitude of risk factors, these tests should be conducted on an annual basis. Medical testing may be considered unwise if you do not wish to have a diagnosis of diabetes or prediabetes stated on your medical charts. A diabetic diagnosis on medical and insurance records can make obtaining health or life insurance a much more costly affair, or may even prevent you from getting these benefits at all. Luckily, it is relatively easy to test yourself at home without any fear of your results being posted to your medical records. This can be achieved by purchasing a low-priced meter to read your blood sugar levels after fasting and post-meals. These meters or test strips do not require a prescription to be purchased.

Diseases Associated with being Overweight

In most instances, a greater BMI rating correlates with a higher risk of suffering from diseases that are associated with being overweight or obese. Diabetes, or excessive blood glucose levels, high blood pressure and arteriosclerosis are all diseases that are included with this correlation. High blood pressure often leads to stroke, kidney damage, heart failure or even retinal damage that causes vision loss. Having high blood pressure also puts you at a greater risk for obtaining diabetes. Arteriosclerosis is a condition that causes the thickening and subsequent narrowing of arteries in the body. This can create coronary and cerebrovascular disorders and is also associated with an increased diabetic risk. High levels of fat within the blood is called hyperlipidemia. This correlates with high cholesterol levels, and as such, is associated as another high risk of obtaining diabetes.

Pets and Diabetes

Diabetes occurs most commonly in household cats and dogs. Those that are deemed middle-aged are typically affected by this disease. It is noted that female dogs are two times as likely to be afflicted as their male counterparts. Some sources state that male cats, on the other hand, are more subject to diabetes than females. However, in both species, all breeds can be affected, though there are certain small dog breeds (such as Miniature Poodles) that have a higher rate of developing diabetes. Symptoms relating to having a diabetic pet can been seen in frequent urination and fluid loss, but the issue is that this disease can also be quite stealthy and symptoms can be overlooked by owners. However, managing diabetic emergencies and keeping up with principles of treatment (weight loss, insulin, oral antidiabetics) are very similar to those in humans. Some other good news is that the long-term complications that humans suffer from this disease are much more rare in animals, though they can suffer from frequent infections.

Statin Drugs and Their Possible Dangers

An estimated amount of an astounding 40 million people take statin drugs every year. The enormous pharmaceutical companies have about a $29 billion reason why they safeguard their continued profits and mislead the general public about facts relating to cholesterol. This is an outrageous amount of money that constitutes for most of the annual profits for pharmaceuticals. Statins easily are the most profitable drugs on our planet. Told from a British medical journal, *NaturalNews*: "To hear Big Pharma tell it, statin drugs are 'miracle' medicines that have prevented millions of heart attacks and strokes." However a study recently published in that same journal tells a different side of the story. What is stated within that study is that for every drug prevented heart attack, there are two or more individuals who suffer from kidney failure, liver damage, extreme muscle weakness or even cataracts as a result of taking these same drugs. Statin drugs seem to certainly cause far more harm for those taking them than what they are intended to help. Only 2.7% of people taking statin drugs actually have these drugs work in their favor while 4.4% of people suffer from serious damages while taking them.

If you are one who takes these statin drugs, the odds of actually having them work for you are less than a 3 out of 100. The odds of being physically harmed by them is greater with a 4 out of 100 chance. For most, statin drugs have little to no benefit to their overall health. The only benefit these drugs are serving is to continually make drug companies more and more money. From large pharmaceutical company views, these drugs also have an additional benefit of creating other conditions and diseases that will often result in the prescription of even more drugs or medical procedures. Kidney dialysis is one of these procedures that has a significant monetary gain for hospitals and serves as a multi-billion-dollar business all on its own.

Statin drugs can simply be viewed as a gateway for the healthcare industry to bring in new patients, especially for kidney dialysis, since a certain percentage of these statin users will inevitably wind up with kidney failure. These medications are a malicious scam that the large pharmaceutical companies have bred into doctors in order to sell more of their highly profiting drugs to people who will likely not even benefit from them anyway. If this truth was more readily known, these same popular drugs would cease to be prescribed to almost everyone. Another heavy reasoning for the large pharmaceutical companies not to tell you this is that they would be sued up into the billions for marketing manipulations, false advertisement and wrongful death. The FDA openly admits to the fact that statin drugs actually can cause diabetes, elevated blood sugar levels, memory loss, muscles damage and liver disease. Basically, the same doctors individuals are depending on to make informative decisions about their health are readily handing out diabetes in a pill form. Medical education has been, and is still, controlled a great deal by large international pharmaceutical organizations in order to continue to protect the mass amount of monetary gain from some of their most profitable drug classes. This education advocates readily handing out these drugs to everyone with the push to even have statins added into the municipal water supplies.

The worldwide spread of diabetes is occurring at epidemic rates and anything that aids in spreading this disease to even more individuals is nothing short of a total catastrophe. This fact, unfortunately, has not halted doctors, who are misinformed about these medications, from passing them out to a number of their patients. What is most interesting is that, for most Americans, the need to worry about high cholesterol is nil, whereas the worry for low cholesterol is a very real issue. Total cholesterol is more important of a number to address as opposed to simply worrying about LDL and HDL levels. If your total cholesterol number is between 200 and 300, you're at a good point! Any lower, and you're at an increased risk for certain types of cancers and hemorrhagic stroke. Doctors and so-called medical experts who have readily given their support of these drugs being handed out at an exponential rate or having them added to the general public's drinking water should really take into account the newest safety data that has been published by the U.S. FDA that states new labeling guidelines for these statin drugs. The risk of getting diabetes, when taking a statin drug, raises up to a whopping 46% (more than double the risk that led to the FDA warning)! Diabetes is caused by these drugs' effects on the body's insulin response by decreasing insulin sensitivity by 24% and insulin secretion by 12%. These factors lead to insulin resistance and what can cause you to become yet another diabetic. If you are already considered diabetic or prediabetic, these symptoms from the disease can be worsened.

Cholesterol is a naturally occurring substance that our bodies produce to be sent to areas where there is inflammation in order to aid with easing the pain. By attacking cholesterol, we are basically taking out the very means by which we help our own bodies. The very problem here is inflammation, not the cholesterol, and it should be looked into as to why the inflammation is being caused and address that. One of the single most prevailing causes of inflammation occurs from taking a daily shower. A typical showerhead will vaporize the chlorine that is in the water and transform that chlorine into a vapor that is then breathed in. This very same chlorine vapor can cause damage to your lungs and arteries, creating inflammation. The solution, however, is simple! If you get an activated charcoal filter that screws on to or above your shower head, it will filter away the chlorine that is contained within the water you're showering with. An even more advantageous solution is to install a "whole house filter" that will eliminate the chlorine and other contaminates that are in the municipal water supply. Chlorine has the capability to bleach your hair along with your laundry, and is a destructive poison that is placed in our water systems in order to kill off pathogens. While it is not in high enough levels to kill people, it still does considerable damage to our bodies. It is advised to filter all chlorine from your cooking water, drinking water and the water that you bathe yourself in. By reducing this exposure to chlorine, you are subsequently reducing inflammation and any need for some of the most profitable drugs - statins.

It is strongly recommended that individuals who are taking the following statin drugs should eliminate exposure to chlorine, become aware of their life-altering side effects and gradually wean themselves off of these medications under the statin category. Regardless of medical conditions (supposed levels of high cholesterol, diabetes, etc.) it is advised to find a doctor who is willing to help you get off of these unnecessary medications: Altoprev (lovastatin ER), Lescol (fluvastatin), Crestor (rosuvastatin), Livalo (pitavastatin), Lipitor (atorvastatin), Pravachol (pravastatin), Zocor (simvastatin), Mevacor (lovastatin), Advicor (lovastatin and niacin ER), Vytorin (simvastatin and ezetimibe) and Simcor (simvastatin and niacin ER).

The Dangers of Insulin

Keeping a watchful eye on glucose levels, diet and exercising can help diabetics lead a long, healthy life. For diabetics, eating nutrient dense foods that are low in carbs, packed with protein and include healthy fats are good health investments. But how exactly does insulin work?

Insulin is a hormone which is produced in the pancreas, and introduced into the bloodstream. It circulates throughout the body, allowing cells access to sugar. Insulin directly lowers levels of sugar in the blood, and as blood sugar drops, insulin levels drop as well. Glucose, a sugar, is the main source of energy, feeding cells of body tissue. It's produced inside of you by your liver and stored in your muscle tissue as glycogen. Glucose is also absorbed by your body from the food that you eat. This sugar is absorbed into the blood, and with the help of insulin, enters cells. If you haven't eaten for a long time, your glucose levels drop. When this happens your liver breaks down the glycogen stored in your muscle tissue back into glucose to moderate your levels, putting them back into a normal range.

Insulin also blocks cholesterol elimination while at the same time delivering cholesterol to arterial cell walls. This results in plaque buildup in the arteries, leading to heart attacks, heart disease and even strokes. For diabetics especially, there is a significant increase in risk for cardiac disease and stroke. Nearly 80% of deaths related to diabetes are due to arterial hardening - mainly of the coronary artery. An increased need for insulin directly results in plaque buildup in the arteries, more so when insulin levels are already at an increased level. Insulin promotes hunger and storage of fats in the body, leading to an increase in body weight, which furthers resistance - resulting in a need for more insulin. Diabetic complications are often a dangerous and deadly spiral for serious cases. Low nutrient processed foods packed with carbs and calories in the Standard American Diet (SAD) only serve to make matters worse. This is definitively harmful to individuals with diabetes. Connections have even been drawn between insulin and cancer. As an example, you are 30% more likely to be diagnosed with colorectal cancer, 20% more likely to develop breast cancer and placed at a staggering 82% increase in risk for pancreatic cancer (the pancreas is where insulin is made). Given the fact that insulin treatment can cause an increase in weight, treating this with more medication to make the pancreas increase its production only makes matters worse. This is a continuing cycle where a diabetic patient requires more insulin because they are gaining weight from insulin in the first place and serves only to make them more sick by causing them to become even more diabetic.

Healthy Supplements

Diabetics, in particular, suffer from a higher level of free radicals in the blood than most other people. This causes oxidative stress on the arteries because of the body's inability to detoxify the blood or reverse the damages caused by the condition. This makes the addition of antioxidants an integral part of diabetes management. Type 1 diabetics will most likely have to be on insulin for the duration of their lifetime. However, by taking supplements to offset complications, a person may be able to reduce the amount of insulin they need and improve their glucose metabolism. Type 2 diabetics may be able to offset the progression of diabetes with antioxidant therapy which will improve their glucose metabolism and improve insulin sensitivity.

There are several antioxidant supplements that have proven effective for diabetic management and blood sugar control.

A notable of these is astaxanthin. This can be found in yeast, microalgae, and many kinds of seafood, such as salmon, krill, crayfish, trout, shrimp, and some crustaceans. In fact, it is the chemical responsible for the pinkish color of salmon and the red color that results when seafood is cooked.

Alpha lipoic acid has positive and beneficial impacts on the effects of diabetes on the body. It not only helps to control blood sugar, but it also has been shown to reduce complications from diabetes, such as kidney and heart disease, as well as diseases prevalent in blood vessels. Alpha lipoic acid helps the body because of its ability to reduce the accumulation of fat. For nearly thirty years in Germany, this supplement has been proven to treat and prevent diabetic neuropathy in patients. Both oral and intravenous doses have reduced symptoms associated with diabetic peripheral neuropathy.

Biotin helps to increase the effectiveness of the enzyme glucokinase in the body, as well as enhancing insulin sensitivity. Glucokinase is responsible in the body for metabolizing glucose in the liver. Diabetics tend to have very low levels of this enzyme in their body.

There is extensive evidence in literature that demonstrates carnitine lowers blood sugar and hemoglobin A1c (HbA1c) levels, increases glucose storage and insulin sensitivity, while also enhancing the metabolic rate of carbohydrates and fat in the body. Type 2 diabetics are particularly prone to carnitine deficiencies.

Diabetics in general have low levels of carnosine in their blood; even a normal, healthy, aging adult loses this as they progress in age. Carnosine is a glycation inhibitor and has been shown to reduce the formation of AGES (advanced glycation end products) and helps to protect against the effects of diabetic neuropathy. Carnosine helps to lower blood sugar, prevents protein cross linking (which can cause cataracts in the eye), and helps to curb inflammation and oxidative stress. Carnosine is helpful for reducing oxidation and glycation of low density lipoprotein (LDL) which may otherwise cause atherosclerosis in diabetics. Blindness is also a concern for many diabetics and carnosine supplements will help to reduce the damage to microscopic blood vessels in the eyes (diabetic retinopathy).

Chromium is a trace mineral that plays a vital role in sugar metabolism. Type 2 diabetics will benefit from chromium supplements in aiding to control blood sugar levels. It will also help metabolize protein, lipids, and carbohydrates. Chromium levels are high in onions, tomatoes, and greens.

Coenzyme Q10 (COQ10) has been shown in multiple studies to control blood sugar, prevent oxidative damages, and lower blood pressure. One study supplemented Type 2 diabetics with 100 mg of COQ10 twice daily. Their HbA1c levels and blood pressure were reduced, demonstrating improved glycemic control in the body. In another study, Type 2 diabetics also showed increased blood flow.

DHEA (dehydroepiandrosterone) improves insulin sensitivity and has shown positive results against obesity. It is not completely understood how DHEA works in the body, but it is thought to improve the way glucose metabolizes in the liver. Animal studies have also shown that B-cells increased in the liver, cells responsible for insulin production. DHEA levels are greatly affected by glucose levels inversely – higher glucose levels produce lower DHEA levels. This hormone is produced in the adrenal gland and can be turned into either estrogen or testosterone by the body. Higher levels of testosterone have been associated with higher insulin sensitivity.

Omega 3 and Omega 6 fatty acids each have benefits when taken as a supplement for diabetics. Omega 3 fatty acids found in marine oil can help to lower triglyceride levels and reduce blood pressure by thinning the blood and reducing inflammation. Omega 6 fatty acid GLA, if given ample time to work in the body, has been shown to slow the progression and severity of diabetic neuropathy, especially when combined with lipoic acid.

Fiber is essential for every human body, but especially so for diabetics because of the effects of long-term elevated blood glucose levels. It's also helpful in controlling the appetite because it makes the person feel full, digests slower, and reduces the urge to snack. Most fibrous foods provide healthy options – ones that are low in fat and high in nutrient content. When experimenting with fibrous foods, it is important to monitor blood sugar and adjust injectable or oral hypoglycemia medications accordingly to account for lower blood glucose levels. The addition of fiber into the diet should be done gradually because intestinal irritation may occur; this can include cramps, bloating, and flatulence.

Propolmannan is a widely used dietary fiber in Asia. It helps to create a barrier in the stomach that significantly reduces the digestion of carbohydrates and slows the process of food moving from the stomach to the small intestine. This helps to safely prevent after-meal blood sugar spikes.

A variety of antioxidants known as flavonoids have been shown to reduce damage caused by diabetes. In some animal studies, the potent flavonoid quercetin reduced blood levels of oxidants and glucose. This particular antioxidant does well in lower doses as it helps to minimize oxidative stress. It also helped to normalize levels of other antioxidants in the body, including Vitamins C and D.

Folic acid and folate are members of the Vitamin B family – folate is found naturally in beans and green vegetables, while folic acid is a synthetic added to vitamins or food supplements. Some evidence suggests that synthetic folic acid may contribute to increased cancer risks, so it is best to stick to the natural folate as a supplement in your diet.

Many diabetics lack magnesium in their bodies because medications tend to deplete this mineral, as well as being furthered by the disease itself. In a double-blind study, the results suggested that adding magnesium supplements to their diet, diabetics were better able to control their blood sugar levels.

Typically used to treat overdoses of acetaminophen, NAC (N-acetylcysteine) has been shown to protect the heart and linings of the blood vessels from damage in diabetic rat studies. One study showed that NAC was able to increase the availability of nitric acid in rats, reducing oxidative stress in their heart tissues and lowering blood pressure.

Silymarin is derived from milk thistle, and in studies among diabetic animals has been shown to improve insulin levels. One small study supplied silymarin daily in 600 mg doses to diabetics who suffered from alcohol-related liver failure. Overall, it was found that the supplement reduced urine and fasting blood glucose levels, after an initial spike during the first month when the users began supplementation. As the blood glucose levels dropped, so too did their HbA1c levels. During the duration of the treatment, fasting glucose levels fell by almost half, resulting in a 24% reduction in daily insulin requirements and improved liver functioning. Also evident were less occurrences of hypoglycemic episodes, which suggests that blood sugar levels were lower *and* had stabilized.

Vitamin B3, also commonly known as niacin, is essential in helping nearly fifty enzymes function within the body. It is responsible for releasing energy to make fat from carbohydrates, as well as making hormones that impact sex drive and other chemicals in the body that trigger signals in the brain. It has been shown in clinical trials to be safe and effective for diabetics. Niacinamide can slow the destruction of and even restore B-cells. Some evidence even suggests that niacin may help to reduce the risk of developing Type 1 diabetes. Because niacin may interrupt diabetics' blood sugar control efforts, any diabetic who supplements with niacin needs to closely monitor their blood sugar levels and discontinue use if control becomes unattainable.

Preclinical studies evaluated the role of Vitamin C during periods of mild oxidative stress. The tissue that surrounds the eye is supplied with Vitamin C through the liquid layers within the eye that provide natural hydration and lubrication between the cornea and the lens. Animal studies have shown that glucose decreases this process of Vitamin C uptake through the eye, resulting in poor functioning in diabetics. Therefore, supplementation of Vitamins C and E as antioxidants can help to improve eye health. High levels of Vitamin C intake have been shown to reduce glycation, providing significant positive consequences in slowing the progression of diabetes. Through the relationship with sorbitol in the body, Vitamin C also prevents ocular degeneration in diabetics by reducing sorbitol buildup. Sorbitol tends to accumulate in the cells of those who suffer from diabetes, which reduces the antioxidant functioning of the eye leading to a number of complications. In a study of diabetics who also suffered from coronary artery disease, Vitamin C supplementation was shown to reduce inflammation and increase blood flow in the body. Combined with other vitamins and minerals, three other studies showed that Vitamin C increases the elasticity of blood vessels, thereby reducing blood pressure and increasing blood flow.

Vitamin D has been known to promote bone health, but studies conducted over the last forty years show other health implications. Animal studies and human observation studies have implied that Vitamin D may help to prevent Type 1 diabetes possibly by strengthening the immune system, preventing certain cytokines from causing attacks on pancreatic cells by the body's autoimmune system. A study of more than 12000 pregnant women in Finland showed protective measures against Type 1 diabetes development in infants. One year into the study, the children who were supplemented with 2000 IU of Vitamin D daily showed lower risks of developing Type 1 diabetes than the children who did not take the supplement. Vitamin D may also slow the loss of insulin sensitivity, reducing susceptibility to Type 2 diabetes in people who have shown early signs of the disease. A three-year study included 314 non-diabetic adults. They were given either a placebo or supplements of 500 mg Calcium and 700 IU of Vitamin D. Those who showed mildly elevated fasting blood glucose levels at the beginning of the study who were given the supplement showed a lower rise in glucose levels during the three-year study than the other subjects who did not take the supplements. The research suggested that, in adults with elevated glucose levels, Vitamin D and Calcium supplementation averted metabolic syndrome and even prevented Type 2 diabetes.

A double-blind study found that Vitamin E helped to reduce damage to the nerves that supply the heart, effectively reducing the risk of cardiac autonomic neuropathy, a common complication in diabetics. Vitamin E also shows evidence for improving blood sugar control, preventing cataracts, and benefits for diabetic peripheral neuropathy. For Type 2 diabetics, Vitamin E enhances insulin sensitivity.

Botanicals and Diabetes

Before the implementation of insulin for control of diabetes, many used botanical supplements because they are safe and effective. However, many botanicals function just as insulin does in the body, so diabetics who use oral medications or insulin need to be aware of dosages to prevent hypoglycemia. When combined with medical advice, exercise, a healthy diet, and other nutritional supplements, botanicals can be an effective diabetes management tool.

A recent study has shown that regularly adding cinnamon to the diet can aid in maintaining a healthy glucose metabolism. The study isolated complexes that enhance insulin production found in cinnamon that help to prevent or alleviate diabetes and glucose intolerance. Three water-soluble polyphenol polymers were found to increase insulin-dependent glucose metabolism by nearly twenty times. These substances also showed significant antioxidant abilities, as did other chemicals found in cinnamon – tannin, phenol, and epicatechin. Long-term use of cinnamon can lead to a buildup of aldehyde compounds, fat-soluble, toxic, and highly reactive substances, however. There is a patented liquid extract of cinnamon that delivers the water-soluble nutrients that are beneficial to the body and at the same time remove fat-soluble toxins from the body. A double-blind study of diabetics with high blood sugar (with a placebo control group) with an average age of 61 years were given 500 mg per day of a cinnamon extract. They averaged a decline of 12 mg/dl in their fasting blood glucose after only two months. Significant to note was the decline of glucose spikes after a meal of 75 grams of carbohydrates by an average of 32 mg/dl. This study correlated with data from other studies using cinnamon extracts in which, after just four months, patients saw an average of a ten percent reduction in their fasting glucose levels.

Another natural way to manage glucose levels involves inhibiting the conversion of starches into sugars in the gastrointestinal tract with the introduction of enzymes that prevent carbohydrates from metabolizing. These inhibitor enzymes can be found in seaweed extracts. Notably, they help to stop alpha-glucosidase and alpha-amylase enzymes which produce sugar in the body. Animal studies showed that inhibiting these specific sugar-producing enzymes lowered overall blood sugar levels. A placebo-controlled double-blind study recently found that supplementation of 500 mg per day of seaweed and bladderwrack in healthy subjects increased insulin sensitivity and resulted in a reduction of postprandial glucose spikes by 48.3%.

African mango (Irvingia gabonensis) extracts have been found to inhibit the conversion of alpha-amylase carbohydrates into sugar. A 1990 study conducted on eleven subjects with Type 2 diabetes found significant reductions in several areas. Total cholesterol was reduced by thirty percent, LDL by thirty-nine percent, blood triglyceride levels fell by sixteen percent, and glucose levels by thirty-eight percent; however, HDL cholesterol levels increased by twenty-nine percent after four weeks. Overall improved clinical health was observed among the subjects experiencing positive biochemical consequences.

Extracts from white kidney beans have shown promising results in human studies, blocking the alpha-amylase enzyme which is beneficial for preventing insulin and blood sugar spikes common with many chronic health problems. In diabetic animals, it has been shown to reduce blood sugar levels by inhibiting the amylase metabolic capabilities. For humans, it also reduces the effects of high glycemic foods, such as white bread, that are responsible for producing dangerous spikes in blood sugar after meals. Phaseolus vulgaris, the common garden bean, has also been shown to reduce postprandial blood sugar spikes by 67%.

Purified and standardized extracts from green coffee beans produce in the body high levels of beneficial polyphenols and chlorogenic acid that reduce excessive blood glucose levels. Roasting coffee beans strips away much of the benefits of the green coffee bean. Chlorogenic acid and caffeic acid are two notable nutrients found in coffee beans that help to manage blood sugar levels. Glucose production from the glycogen stored in the liver tends to be overactive in people with high blood sugar. An enzyme critical to regulating blood sugar, glucose-6-phosphatase, if reduced, can lead to overall reduced blood sugar levels. In one study, researchers provided varying dosages of chlorogenic acid-standardized green coffee bean extract to fifty-six subjects. Thirty-five minutes later, the subjects orally ingested 100 grams of glucose. As the test dosages of extract increased from 200 mg to 400 mg, the reduction in blood sugar levels decreased significantly, markedly by a 24% reduction with the 400 mg dose.

Garlic and onions contain an active ingredient called allium that provides sulfur for a vital internal antioxidant process. Allium has many positive implications for reducing diabetic complications such as cardiovascular disease and atherosclerosis, decreasing oxidative stress, lowering blood pressure, helping in weight loss, improving insulin sensitivity, and improving cholesterol.

Green tea has always been known to have powerful antioxidant properties. Catechin, epigallocatechin, epicatechin, and gallocatechin are especially powerful in reducing toxins in the liver and pancreas. Some animal studies suggest that gallocatechin has been shown to prevent diabetes. In rat studies, this antioxidant prevented B-cell destruction caused by cytokine by decreasing the amount of nitric oxide synthase in the body, a pro-oxidant, which may help slow the progression of Type 1 diabetes. In vitro studies have also demonstrated that green tea can help suppress obesity caused by diet, which is a risk factor in the development of metabolic syndrome and diabetes.

In studies conducted on diabetic rats, ginkgo biloba was shown to prevent diabetic retinopathy. One clinical trial provided Type 2 diabetic adults with an oral ginkgo biloba supplement for three months. Their levels of free radicals were reduced, fibrinogen levels dropped, and blood viscosity improved. In patients with retinopathy, extracts of ginkgo improved capillary blood flow as well. Ginkgo has been observed to reduce blood glucose levels in a study of Type 2 diabetics over the course of three months when supplemented with 120 mg per day. Liver metabolism of insulin and orally ingested hypoglycemic medications improved, reducing plasma glucose levels. Those who benefited most from ginkgo supplements were Type 2 diabetics suffering from pancreatic exhaustion. It does not appear that ginkgo biloba improves the production of beta cells, but merely allows the liver more efficiency in metabolizing existing insulin levels.

Blueberries are native to North America and have been used in many foods, as well as for therapeutic purposes because of their antioxidant properties. Scientists attribute their antioxidant strengths to polyphenols called anthocyanins. In Type 2 diabetic patients, blueberries reduced baseline blood sugar levels by 37%.

Diabetic rat studies demonstrated that bilberry reduced their vascular permeability, and mice receiving bilberry-containing herbal extracts showed significantly lower blood sugar levels. A placebo-controlled double-blind study of fourteen diabetics suffering from retinopathy who took bilberry extract supplements showed promising improvements early in the day after blood testing. There were also other open trials in humans that showed the benefits of bilberry.

It is never advisable to discontinue diabetic drug therapy – especially insulin – without consulting a doctor. However, blood glucose metabolism can be improved by supplementing with the suggested amounts of the following:

- COQ10 (in the form of ubiquinol): 100 to 300 mg daily
- DHEA: 15 – 75 mg
- EPA/DHA: 1400 mg EPA and 1000 mg DHA daily
- Fiber (guar, pectin, propolmannan, or oat bran): 20 to 30 g
- Propolmannan: 2 grams twice daily

- Astaxanthin: 4000 mg daily at least (up to 50 g daily)
- R-lipoic acid: 240 – 480 mg daily
- L-carnitine: 500 – 1000 mg twice daily
- Carnosine: 500 mg twice daily
- Quercetin: 500 mg daily
- Chromium: 500 – 1000 mcg daily
- Magnesium: 140 mg daily as magnesium L-threonate; or 320 mg daily as magnesium citrate
- NAC: 500 – 1000 mg daily
- Silymarin: containing 750 mg Silybum marianum (standardized to 80 percent Silymarin, 30 percent Silibinin, and 8% Isosilybin A and Isosilybin B)
- Vitamin C: at least 2000 mg daily
- Vitamin E: 400 IU daily (with 200 mg gamma tocopherol)
- GLHC: 1200 mg daily
- Green tea extract: 725 mg green tea extract (minimum 93% polyphenols)
- Ginkgo biloba: 120 mg daily
- Bilberry extract: 100 mg daily
- B complex: Containing the entire B family, including biotin and niacin
- Cinnamon extract: 175 mg (Cinnamomum cassia) standardized to 2.5% (4.375 mg) A-type polymers three times daily
- Green coffee bean extract: 200 – 400 mg (standardized to contain chlorogenic acid) three times a day
- Vitamin D3: 2000 – 5000 IU daily

- Brown seaweed and bladderwrack: 100 mg three times per day
- Irvingia gabonensis: 150 mg twice a day
- White kidney bean: 445 mg twice a day
- Blueberry: standardized to contain 50 mg 3,4-chlorogenic acid, and 50 mg myricetin; or 22.5 g blueberry bioactive freeze dried powder
- Folate: best obtained from greens and beans

Stress and Health

It has always been accepted knowledge that stress is harmful to the body, to the point of contributing to death in extreme cases, but recent scientific research has proven *why* stress can lead to death. Stress has been shown to cause the body's cells to shut down. When cells begin to close down, they are not able to take in nutrients, causing them to become weakened, susceptible to disease, and eventually die. This explains the reason that two people can have the same disease, but one will be able to recover while the other will continue to decline in health and possibly die. When the body is stressed, healthy cells cannot absorb the proper nutrients they need to thrive and fight disease.

Even in instances where there is ample internal insulin to promote absorption of blood sugar into the cells, under stress the cells simply cannot receive the sugars they need to function. This causes blood glucose blockage from entering cells, resulting in high blood glucose and insulin resistance – the medical definition of diabetes. The cells fail to respond to insulin produced by the pancreas. All forms of stress can cause blood sugar to become uncontrollable, which is especially dire for someone who already has been diagnosed with diabetes, those with undiagnosed diabetes (since they don't know they need help controlling their blood sugar), or those who show early signs of diabetes.

Weakened cells become easy targets for infection and disease including cancerous cells. Under stress, the body's blood sugar rises, even in healthy individuals without prediabetic symptoms or a full diabetic diagnosis. Stress causes the body to release cortisol and epinephrine hormones to increase energy levels, which they achieve by increasing the level of blood sugar in the body. Stress also causes the risk of developing cardiovascular diseases, heart attacks, or stroke. By decreasing the factors that cause stress, it will allow cells in the body to become receptive to the nutrition they need to be healthy and fight off diseases and ailments, including diabetes.

The body can thrive when the cells are able to receive what they need. Even in individuals with diseases or illnesses already present in the body, lowering stress levels will allow the cells to become healthier and stronger, making them better able to fight the disease. For individuals without disease, the cells are able to resist diseases from becoming established in the body.

Stress is like a chemical disaster for the body. It causes a flood of catabolic hormones that have destructive tendencies. These hormones, like cortisol, cause the body to store fat especially in the middle (belly) area, which is an indicator of early diabetes. There is a high number of receptor sites in fat cells in this area of the body that are sensitive to cortisol and leptin, another fat-sensitive hormone. These hormones can also contribute to anxiety, depression, and other emotional instabilities that cause a person to drastically change their diets. Emotional eating causes a person to lose sight of maintaining a healthy diet and they tend to eat more fat, carbohydrates, and sugars than is normal or healthy. Diabetics need to stick to a low-carb diet and not let stress and emotional eating get them off track.

Stress is a severely impacting factor on cardiovascular health and causes more heart attacks than regular, healthy exercise. Stress is a contributing factor in nearly every disease – literally, a lack of ease. The immune system is suppressed by emotional stress, and chronic elevated stress levels lead to diseases. Extreme and on-going instances of fight or flight stress can have long-term, lasting effects. Digestion slows down, inhibiting metabolism which affects the immune system. Stress is detrimental to maintain healthy cholesterol levels. Shallow or rapid breathing, muscle tension, and increased heart rate and blood pressure are also signs of stress. Blood flow is restricted and stress inhibits the body's ability to heal itself.

Personality types can also affect the way a person deals with stress. Dominant or hostile and aggressive personalities cause the person to be susceptible to more stressors leading to disease. Hostile personalities tend to experience higher levels of stress and these individuals are three to four times more likely to develop diseases and die at younger ages. Personalities with low hostile tendencies experience less stress, and overall less adverse health effects. Being involved in angry or hostile relationships can cause undue stress on the body.

Everyone is capable of experiencing stress. While minor stress or experiencing stress in a healthy way can make a person more efficient under some circumstances, there is a point the body reaches where it no longer becomes efficient. Listening to relaxing music, visualization, breathing exercises, and meditation help the body to relax, reducing stress, lowering heart rate and blood pressure, easing muscle tension, and enhancing the immune system. Here are some other ways to purposely reduce stress and the overall negative effects it may have on the body:

- Smile and laugh often
- Speak powerful words softly
- Reduce or eliminate the use of cell phones and other electronics
- Take breaks at work
- Avoid reading or watching too much news
- Engage in hobbies or activities you enjoy often
- Plant a garden
- Adopt a pet
- Do one random act of kindness a day
- Have more sex
- Get out of debt
- Don't drive while talking on the phone
- Be thankful
- Use aromatherapy
- Get rid of your alarm clock

Most people start their day with the sound of an alarm clock jolting them from their sleep. This isn't the body awakening, but rather a shocking of the brain into an awakened state which releases stress hormones. Starting the day with a dose of stress hormones coursing through the blood is not the way to go. It is healthier to wake slowly and gently. There are alarm clocks that use gentle tones or sounds of nature to wake a person out of sleep. They start at a lower volume and gradually get louder as it goes off. Making this small change can improve your emotional state and even balance the body's pH level.

By reducing stress at home and at work, you will become more efficient and happier. Physical stress, emotional, financial and all other types of stress should be evaluated. Remember that stress isn't just something you feel – it is a chemical explosion in the body, causing damages you don't feel and can't see – ultimately leading to or worsening a disease, including diabetes, and even death. By flipping the stress switch to "off" and flipping "on" the good health switch you will allow your body to experience optimal health benefits and it will be able to heal itself at the cellular level. Your cells will be able to absorb the nutrients they need to thrive – oxygen, sugar, water – which will result in healing from the inside out.

Holmes and Rahe Stress Scale

Holmes and Rahe's Stress Scale is a list of stressful events (with assigned Life Change Units) that can lead to or contribute to illness. To find a 'score' is to add up the Life Change Units associated with events a person has experienced during the course of the past year. The score gives an estimate of how stress can affect one's health. Based on a person's age, there are two different tables that may apply: Adults and Non-Adults. The total Life Change Units score and the associated effects are the same.

Scoring Scale:

- 300+ Life Change Units: At risk of developing illness
- 150-299 Life Change Units: Moderate risk of illness (30% decrease from risk with 300+ Life Change Unit score)
- <150 Life Change Units: Slight risk of illness

ADULTS

Life Event	Life Change Units
Death of a Partner/Spouse	100
Divorce	73
Marital Separation	65
Jail term	63
Personal injury	53
Marriage	50
Fired from work	47
Marital reconciliation	45
Retirement	45
Change in family member's health	44
Pregnancy	40
Sexual difficulties	39
Addition to family	39
Business readjustment	39
Change in financial status	38
Death of close friend	37
Change in work	36

Change in amount of marital arguments	35
Mortgage/loan of >$10,000	31
Foreclosure	30
Change in responsibilities at work	29
Child leaving home	29
Trouble with in-laws	29
Outstanding personal achievement	28
Spouse enters/leaves workforce	26
Starting/finishing school	26
Change in living conditions	25
Revision of personal habits	24
Trouble with boss	23
Change in work conditions/hours	20
Change in residence	20
Change in schools	20
Change in recreational habits	19
Change in religious activities	19
Change in social activities	18
Mortgage/loan of <$10,000	17
Change in sleeping habits	16
Change in number of family gatherings	15
Change in eating habits	15
Vacations	13
Christmas season	12
Minor violation of the law	11

NON-ADULTS

Life Event	Life Change Units
Death of a parent	100
Unplanned pregnancy/abortion	100
Getting married	95
Parents divorcing	90

Acquiring a physical deformity	80
Fathering a child	70
Jail sentence of parent (>one year)	70
Parents separation	69
Death of sibling	68
Change in acceptance by peers	67
Sister's unplanned pregnancy	64
Discovery of being adopted	63
Marriage of parent to step-parent	63
Having visible congenital deformity	62
Serious illness requiring hospitalization	58
Failure of a grade in school	56
Not making extracurricular activity	55
Hospitalization of a parent	55
Jail sentence of parent (>30 days)	53
Breaking up with boyfriend or girlfriend	53
Beginning to date	51
School suspension	50
Becoming involved with drugs or alcohol	50
Birth of a sibling	50
Increase in parents' arguments	47
Loss of job by parent	46
Outstanding personal achievement	46
Change in parent's financial status	45
Accepted at college of choice	43
Being a high school senior	42
Hospitalization of a sibling	41
Increased absence of parent from home	38
Sibling leaving home	37
Addition of third adult to family	34
Becoming a full church member	31
Decrease in arguments between parents	26
Decrease in arguments with parents	26
Parent beginning to work	26

Light's Effect on Eyesight and Sleep

Are you aware that LED screens have a huge impact on how efficient our sleep cycle is? The importance of sleep is vital for everyone, but this is especially true for those with diabetes. A danger lies within the very devices we use on a daily basis. Computers, cell phones and a number of other electronic devices harbor a spectrum of light that can greatly affect our eyesight and sleep pattern.

Throughout the day, the color temperature of computer screens appeals to our eyes because they are designed to replicate daylight emitted from the sun. Once the sun sets, however, it's probably best not to continue with these same daylight color temperatures. Ever notice that "blue halo" or "eerie blue glow" an individual is illuminated with when in front of a computer screen at night? Have you ever been blinded by your computer screen when you awake and go to the computer to jot down your ideas? Have you ever experienced trouble falling asleep or even staying asleep after spending great lengths of time staring at an LED computer screen? In 2012, the American Medical Association (AMA) released a report from its Council on Science and Public Health that recommended: "Recognize that exposure to excessive light at night, including extended use of various electronic media, can disrupt sleep or exacerbate sleep disorders, especially in children and adolescents." So, what are blue and ultraviolet light and what are their effects on our bodies?

Blue light is a part of the light spectrum that we, as humans, experience. It is emitted by artificial light sources, such as LED computer screens and smartphones, as well as by the sun. There are certain kinds of blue light that are advantageous by helping with the regulation of the body's natural internal clock. This same blue light, however, can also have negative impacts on our eyes, especially in reference to the retina. This light is also a factor of risk for the onset of age-related macular degeneration. This affects the portion of the retina that controls sharpness and centralized vision.

Ultraviolet light, on the other hand, is not within our visible light spectrum. It is most noted for its ability to increase skin cancer risks but it is also considerably detrimental for our eyes. Without the proper protection, excess exposure to ultraviolet light can wind up producing cataracts. Photokeratitis, or sunburn of the eye's cornea, is another possibility that can contribute to interim blindness. Because of these risks, it's a valid question as to whether we should be protecting ourselves against the ultraviolet and blue light that emanates from the conglomerate of electronics we obtain. This includes our laptops, tablets and cell phones.

A study conducted recently discovered that Americans spend around 2 ½ hours of their day on their smartphones and tablets. As such, it is crucial that any individual using digital devices on such a consistent basis protect themselves against this light emission. Yet, it's not only these devices that originate blue light. Fluorescent light bulbs and LEDs are used by most stores and offices due to their energy efficiency. The importance of safeguarding your eyes from this exposure matters not only indoors but outdoors as well.

Even on the cloudiest of days, our eyes are exposed to ultraviolet radiation. We are actually exposed to up to 40% of ultraviolet light when out of full sunlight. Ultraviolet light can make its way indoors through our windows. For those who are in their cars quite often or stay close to windows in their home or office, this can be a particularly hazardous fact. There are a number of people who are at great risk for daily overexposure of both ultraviolet and blue light. Understanding some of the risks of this light exposure is pertinent, but how does blue light affect our sleep?

It is already known that blue light has a tendency to keep individuals up later than they may want to be. LED screens that emit this blue light can potentially injure your eyes because of the UVB lighting that is within this blue light spectrum. Research has shown that individuals may find that their sleep is hindered by about an hour if they engage with an LED television, computer screen or tablet a few hours before going to bed. There is a high likelihood that you are simply not getting your required amount of sleep due to your television, cell phone, tablet or computer. Luckily, there is a free software you can download, called f.lux, that alters the coloration temperature of your computer screen to match the time of day the device is used. This software also works for a number of tablets and smartphones. The adaptation between daylight and warm lighting in the evening can allow the user to experience a better night's sleep. Some individuals simply use f.lux because they feel that it makes the overall appearance of their computer better. This software allows your screen to match the room you're in at all times. Once the sun sets, f.lux makes your device alter to your indoor lighting. Then, once the morning comes around again, it switches the device's lighting to appear as daylight. One must simply inform f.lux of the type of lighting you have in your house and where you reside. That's it! The rest is all automatically done by f.lux. This free software is recommended for everyone but is particularly essential for those who spend a majority of their time in front of a computer screen, especially if a good amount of that time is spent while the sun is down. Why not give it a go? As another recommendation, speak with your ophthalmologist about computer glasses that block UVB rays and that are optimized for your computer viewing distance as opposed to a regular reading distance.

Elements of Diabetic Blood

The most concerning long-term complications of diabetes are in relation to blood vessel damage resulting from blood clots. Those with diabetes are subject to blood clots due to abnormal thickness with their platelets. They also have a tendency to have blood that contains higher levels of fibrinogen, a type of protein. Fibrinogen is essential to all bodies since it clots the blood. Without this clotting protein, a simple paper cut could result in fatality. Though, when an individual has too much of this protein, it can result in the blood becoming too "sticky" or thick which subsequently causes clots to form quite readily. Diabetics also have a tendency to show higher levels of numerous other blood proteins that promote coagulation. This will cause blood clots to form at random within capillaries and the coronary arteries. These blood clots cause about 75% of diabetic fatalities due to the damage that the major arteries suffer, subsequently resulting in strokes and heart attacks. Complications that are most prevalent in diabetics are caused by blood clots within miniscule capillaries. The body's kidneys, eyes, nerves and pancreas are often what are damaged from these capillary clots. High blood pressure is yet another risk diabetes can cause and is another contributing factor for both stroke and heart disease.

Low doses of aspirin, or other medications that thin the blood, have been historically prescribed by conventional doctors. However, more recent studies have shown that these drugs do nothing to address the blood stickiness and are no longer recommended for treatment. The necessity is in making the blood platelets "slippery" again in order to avert death or bodily harm caused by the blood cells clotting too readily. There is a means by which to obtain more "slippery" blood within your veins, though. It is a manner that is also superior at transferring glucose and oxygen to our cells. At no extra cost, this process is also beneficial to those in need of blood because of surgery, blood disorders or injury. Simply put, you donate your blood to local hospitals or blood banks on a regular basis. Now, how does becoming a blood donor help if you are diabetic?

Typically, women harbor about 8-10 pints of blood, men have about 10-12 pints and children under the age of 13 have about 8 pints or lower. When the body creates new red blood cells they are slippery and flexible and they stay in circulation for 100 to 120 days before they are recycled by the body's white blood cells in a process known as macrophage. When red blood cells age they lose flexibility, increasing their stickiness. This increase in blood thickness means that the body has a higher probability of creating blood clots. Subsequently, the red blood cells also lose efficiency with their main job - delivering oxygen to the body's cells. When an individual donates blood, that person rids their body of some of their older, sticky red blood cells. This then forces the body to replenish them with new, flexible and slippery blood cells that are much less likely to create clotting issues. There is also the matter of the reduction of recycling load on macrophage. The macrophage process rids the body of diseased cells, cellular debris and dead or dying cells. Though, in freeing the white blood cells from this process, they can then go about their essential duties of contributing to the body's immune system. The new red blood cells are much more efficient at transferring oxygen to cells so that they can then burn glucose that will fuel the body. This can actually help to improve insulin resistance in diabetics. It's also possible to triple the production of red blood cells for a full hour by jumping up and down for two minutes using a rebounder.

The Future of the Bionic Pancreas

There is an arising prospect for individuals with Type 1 diabetes - the "bionic pancreas". It automatically imitates the tasks of an actual pancreas by delivering both the insulin needed to lower blood sugar and the glucagon to raise it. For the percentage of Type 1 diabetics who have a pancreas that produces absolutely no insulin, this could potentially improve the management of blood sugar by a significant amount. Insulin management isn't the only advantageous possibility. To combat the threat of an opposite condition of having too low of blood sugar, glucagon management is another hope. Most Type 1 diabetics find it nearly impossible to participate in sports or other prolonged physical activities because arduous exercise can be a trigger for hypoglycemic episodes where their blood sugar levels become dangerously low. The result of hypoglycemia can be coma or even death. However, Type 1 diabetics could participate in exercise regimens or sports activities with the use of a bionic pancreas due to its ability to stabilize blood sugar. Basically, this device works by combining the technology of a smartphone, a continuous glucose monitor and a dual pump that enables the proper delivery of hormones into the bloodstream as they are needed. Though all these components have been available on their own for quite some time, together they work in an automated system that can be utilized within a "real world" environment in order to have a continued observation of blood sugar levels. A body that regulates itself normally responds to a drop in blood sugar by secreting glucagon. In the opposite instance, the body will supply insulin when blood sugar reaches too high a level. However, a diabetic's body doesn't have this luxury. With the bionic pancreas, the same response would be done automatically, without testing. The "brain" of this bionic pancreas would be the smartphone, where information regarding blood sugar levels is sent. Then, every five minutes, the smartphone, via Bluetooth wireless connectivity, instructs how much glucagon or insulin the pumps need to deliver. All calculations and guesswork, originally conducted by the patient, is taken out of the equation with this device. If interested in learning more about this device, search for "TEDx bionic pancreas" with Google's search engine.

Perils of Diet

Unfortunately, even friends and family don't always have the best intentions when they push unhealthy or potentially dangerous food and drink items on those with diabetes. It is crucial for diabetic individuals to stay even-headed when having to deal with these types of people while on their journey to achieve a healthier lifestyle. Those who have malicious intent to sabotage healthy eating plans are often envious that they, themselves, do not have the commitment, determination or simply the information in order to do the same for themselves or to respect a good diabetic diet. It may be hard, but be sympathetic because it helps us achieve what is wanted in return - that same sympathy and compassion. When possible, respond with statements that do not describe them, but describe you. By keeping a more positive outlook, you can avoid situations where you could wind up offending others or attacking them because you are upset. There are certain situations where you will encounter others who are negative towards anything that you choose to say or do in regards to your nutrition. Simply avoid talking to them about healthy eating habits and continue on with positive nutritional actions. Let your health results speak for themselves.

If you choose to occasionally enjoy a meal that is not a part of your regular meal plan, know that this is not going to ruin your efforts. In fact, this can actually be a refreshing break from your routine. A toxic thought is that one bad meal will offset your healthy lifestyle completely and is reason to give up on your healthy goals. So, go ahead - make your grandmother smile by enjoying some of her infamous cooking, just keep your portions small and don't overdo it. With the coming days, you can continue onward with your healthy food plan, and remember, don't get yourself upset over a break in your plans.

Avoiding Free Radicals

There are highly reactive, harmful molecules that attack the membranes of cells, proteins and even our very DNA. These molecules are called free radicals. They can speed up the process of aging, weaken our immune system, cause our cells to breakdown and also promote an enormous range of disease that includes cancer, dementia and heart disease. These risks are especially elevated for those with diabetes. Our bodies actually produce these free radicals as a normal metabolic function, so it is impossible to avoid them completely. However, by taking in fewer and healthier calories, once can reduce their overall exposure. Simply by avoiding the consumption of rancid oil and eating a diet that is more plant-based, you can avoid taking in extra free radicals. Plant-based diets contain phytonutrients, which are chemical components that reduce the damage of free radicals. These can be found in white tea, green tea, Vitamin E, Vitamin C, Selenium, Astaxanthin, CoQ10, Zinc and foods that have high ORAC values or a high antioxidant content.

What are Antioxidants?

Free radicals can be deactivated by antioxidants. Kale, blueberries, strawberries, concord grape, spinach, cinnamon and clove are all prosperous sources of antioxidants. The following are some compounds, vitamin precursors, vitamins, minerals and cofactors that aid in the destruction of free radicals:

B Vitamins - This category has numerous vitamins within it that include B1 (thiamine), B2 (riboflavin), B3 (niacin), B6 (pyridoxine), B9 (folate) and B12 (a natural methylcobalamin form). Together, they form what is known as the Vitamin B Complex. These vitamins have been noted as being antioxidant cofactors, meaning they play a supportive role in allowing the list of subsequent antioxidants to work in a more effective manner.

Beta Carotene - This must be present for Vitamin A to be formed by the body as it is a precursor to Vitamin A. Leafy greens, pumpkin, squash, carrots, sweet potatoes, yams, broccoli, peaches, cantaloupes, apricots and a type of seaweed called nori are all incredible sources of beta carotene.

Vitamin C - The most superlative sources for this water-soluble vitamin are citrus fruits. Oranges, lemons, grapefruit and limes are all carriers, as well as tomatoes, strawberries, broccoli, Brussels sprouts, leafy greens, acerola berries and green peppers.

Vitamin E - This is a fat-soluble vitamin with sources from dried beans, other legumes, whole grains, eggs and leafy greens.

Carotenoids - These are fat-soluble antioxidants that increase numbers of lymphocytes (white blood cells) and other natural killer cells in the body. The best sources of carotenoids come from fruits and vegetables, such as tomatoes, kale, carrots, cantaloupes and other red and yellow vegetables.

Zinc - This is yet another essential antioxidant cofactor. Zinc is a mineral that aids with your immune system. An average individual needs between 20 to 50 mg daily. Higher doses can actually inhibit immune functions. You typically do not require zinc supplements as whole grains and meats are excellent sources of this mineral.

Iron - There is a delicate balance with iron since a shortage can increase your potential for infection because it can weaken numerous types of immune cells, however too much iron can also hinder your body's immune function. For women who are of childbearing age, a daily dose of 15 mg is needed. Men require 10 mg of iron daily. Good sources of iron include beans, tofu and meats, but iron supplementation is advantageous if your body is deficient in iron. There are actually a large number of women who are iron deficient because of blood loss that occurs while menstruating. Most individuals do not realize that coffee actually inhibits iron absorption, so it is wise to have your iron levels monitored if you are an avid coffee drinker and especially so if you also happen to be a woman who is premenopausal.

Selenium - This is another immensely powerful antioxidant cofactor that promotes immune cell growth and stimulates antibody production. There are quite a few people who are deficient in this mineral, but you can find it within nuts, seeds, whole grains and seafood. Selenomax yeast is another great source.

Coenzyme Q10 (CoQ10) - These supplements are especially advantageous in the fight against free radicals. CoQ10 is crucial for our health but is not readily available within our food sources. Since CoQ10 decreases in amount with age, a supplemental dose of 150 to 200 mg is recommended if you are 30 years old or greater.

Astaxanthin - This is a substance that is more recently discovered and is an amazingly powerful antioxidant. Salmon and wild shrimp harbor astaxanthin in small amounts, however the best source is in krill oil. Krill oil is harvested from small Antarctic shrimp, and the very best is Neptune Krill Oil which is produced by a patented process.

It has been shown in a recent study that the most common antioxidants can actually aid our bodies in the fight against some of the most rampant health issues that we deal with today. In one placebo-controlled study, Israeli researches provided 70 patients from their hypertension (high blood pressure) clinic with either a combination of antioxidants or a placebo. The dosages of the antioxidants were: Vitamin C (1,000 mg per day), vitamin E (400 IU per day), CoQ10 (120 mg per day) and selenium (200 mcg per day). Patients were then tested at three months and again when at six months. In both instances, the patients who had been given the antioxidant supplements had improved blood sugar levels and control. They had lower blood pressure and also showed significant increases in HDL cholesterol (good cholesterol). They also showed an improvement in the health of their arteries.

What Is An ORAC Chart?

You may have heard about how antioxidants are great for your body. ORAC is the abbreviation of Oxygen Radical Absorbance Capacity.

It's a way of finding out how many antioxidants a food item has. The higher the number, the more antioxidants – simple, right?

For example, cinnamon is way up high in the charts with a value with 267,536. You can imagine what an antioxidant effect it has when you add it in your food.

Add some in your oatmeal, or into your tea. Not only do you get the spicy cinnamon aroma, but you also benefit from its antioxidant properties.

Dark chocolate and milk chocolate, on the other hand, have lower values of 20,823 and 7,528, respectively. What did we want to exemplify with this? Well, it's that if you're going to eat chocolate – make it dark.

Vegetables such as raw broccoli have an ORAC count of 1,362. Does that mean you should replace broccoli with dark chocolate? Of course not. The antioxidants in broccoli serve other purposes. For example, did you know that they can be useful for cancer patients?

We also wanted to prove that dark chocolate does have some neat health benefits. Now, when we say dark, we mean chocolate with an over 70% cacao ratio. If you can, look for alternative with little to no sugar and additive content.

The purer the cacao, the higher the flavonoid content is in the chocolate. Red wine and green teas are also great ways to obtain flavonoids, although cacao is much better in that regard.

How do flavonoids help? Well, they boost both platelet and endothelial function. In short, flavonoids enforce the cell lining of your veins and arteries.

This means your blood flow is improved all around. You heard that right – dark chocolate (in moderation) helps you out with your blood pressure! Bet you didn't think you were going to read that in your lifetime, eh?

Want More Antioxidants? Diversify Your Menu

The one thing you need to know about ORAC amounts is that spices are the most potent in that respect. Next come dried fruits, although you should watch out for the high sugar content.

Due to the fact that there is no water in them, the ORAC value is about 2 to 3 times higher in dried fruit than raw ones.

You can create a nutritional and healthy snack out of just a handful of dried fruit. Mix in a bunch of dried cranberries, nuts, and cherries, and you have a raw meal that's tasty, nutritious and rich in ORAC.

Cooked vegetables are also great for this purpose. For example, if you cook red cabbage you get an ORAC count of 3,145. On the other hand, the raw veggie itself only has a value of 2,252.

You remember broccoli's value was placed at 1,362. Well, if you cook it, you get an ORAC of 2,386.

Here is a more detailed list of ORAC values per 100g of each item:

- Orange 1,819
- Dried Apples 6,681
- Fuji Apple 2,589
- Apricots, raw 1,115
- Apricots, dried 3,234
- Pear, raw 2,941
- Pear, dried 9,496
- Chokeberry, raw 15,820
- Cranberries, 9,584
- Broccoli, raw 1,362
- Broccoli, cooked 2,386
- Red Cabbage, raw 2,252
- Red Cabbage, cooked 3,145
- Artichokes, cooked 9,416
- Dark Chocolate 20,823
- Milk Chocolate 7,528
- Peanuts 3,166
- Almonds 4,454
- Hazelnuts 9,645
- Pecans, 17,940
- Walnuts 13,541
- Brazil Nuts, 4,805
- Ginger Root, 14,840
- Chili powder 23,636
- Marj oram, fresh 27,297
- Thyme, fresh 27,426
- Black pepper 27,618

- Ginger, ground 28,811
- Mustard seed, yellow 29,257
- Sage, fresh 32,004
- Chocolate, Dutched powder 40,200
- Curry Powder 48,504
- Baking Chocolate, unsweetened 49,926
- Basil, dried 67,553
- Parsley, dried 74,349
- Cumin seed 76,800
- Cocoa, dry powder, unsweetened 80,933
- Turmeric, ground 159,277
- Dried Oregano 200,129
- Ground Cinnamon 267,536
- Ground Cloves 314,446

It's probably easier to gauge the ORAC values if we present them per typical serving, rather than for 100g. After all, not everyone has a kitchen scale to weigh their food all the time. Here's a helpful list:

- Apples, Red Delicious, raw, without skin, 1 med 4,727
- Blueberries, raw, 1/2 cup 4,848
- Apples, Golden Delicious, raw, with skin, 1 med 4,859
- Plums, black diamond, with peel, raw, 1 fruit 5,003
- Nuts, pecans 1 oz 5086
- Candies, semisweet chocolate, 1 oz 5,118
- Apples, Gala, raw, with skin, 1 med 5,147
- Prune juice, canned, 1 cup 5,212
- Pears, raw, one med 5,235

- Cranberries, raw, 1/2 cup 5,271
- Apples, raw, with skin, 1 med 5,609
- Artichokes, boiled, 1/2 med 5,650
- Alcoholic drink, wine, table, red, 5 fl oz. 5,693
- Plums, dried (prunes), uncooked, 1/2 cup 5,700
- Candies, chocolate, dark, 1 oz 5,903
- Juice, Pomegranate, 100%, 1 cup 5,923
- Apples, Granny Smith, raw, with skin, 1 med 7,094
- Apples, Red Delicious, raw. with skin, 1 med 7,781
- Elderberries, raw. 1/2 cup 10,655
- Baking chocolate, unsweetened, 1 square 14,479

What You Need to Know About Raw Food

Raw foods contain enzymes that help out the digestive process. Besides being rich in valuable nutrients, that is.

Sprouts, for example, are fantastic sources of nutrition. The best part about them and seeds, is that you can grow them yourself, right at home. Fresh food for the whole family!

Speaking of freshness – you should know that cooked food has a vastly lower amount of vitamins and nutrients than raw food.

Keep the vegetable cooking to a minimum if you want to gain the most out of your diet. If you must cook them, just give them a light steam or a quick sauté.

Raw veggies cooked at temperatures above 118 degrees are deprived of essential enzymes. By destroying these enzymes, you force your body to produce its own.

As such, you consume much more energy to digest food, leaving you open to chronic illness. By leaving the veggies firm to the touch, you preserve at least some part of the nutrients.

When it comes to other foods, you can just steam or blanch them. Grab a food thermometer and make sure your cooked food doesn't pass the 118 degrees threshold.

Also, you should make sure to get organically grown veggies and fruits. Grocery store items are usually filled with plenty of harmful substances.

Plus, they're usually grown in soil that's very poor in nutrients. You could eat twice as much and it still wouldn't yield the same nutritional value – or even mouth-watering flavor – as organically grown food.

We have a great tip for you as well: don't mix raw and cooked food. Your stomach acid levels will rise and you'll just get a bad case of indigestion.

Eating your food raw lets you digest it much faster – almost 2 to 3 times faster, in fact. On the other hand, cooked or canned food just overworks your organs, especially the pancreas.

You could even lose the ability to properly digest things in your old age. Keep in mind what we told you about how to cook your food, and you should be fine.

Great Snacks: Nuts and Seeds

Nuts and seeds make for awesome snacks in-between meals if you don't want to overstuff yourself. Just make sure they're organically grown, and raw. Remember what we said about cooking?

You could even sprout your own crops to gain the maximum amount of nutrients. Or, if you're the buying type, get them while they're still in their shell for the same effect.

The Golden Benefits of Sprouts

As was discussed so far, fresh food holds the key to a nutrient-rich diet. Sprouts have plenty of those, and helpful antioxidants and digestive enzymes as well.

You can basically just sprout nuts, seeds, and beans in fresh water at home, and you're growing your own organic meals.

Furthermore, you get a necessary increase in vitamins and minerals, while lowering your carbs and caloric intake in the process.

Let's offer a concrete example in the form of mung beans. Here's what you get from freshly grown beans vs. dried ones:

- A 15% decrease in both caloric and carb content – lots of carbs are broken down during the sprouting process.

- 30% more protein availability – this gives you a hint of how much more nutritional organically sprouted food is;
- 34% more Calcium -
- 80% more Potassium;
- 690% more Sodium – which is crucial for removing carbon dioxide and aiding in digestion (along with the vitamin increase shown below);
- 40% more Iron;
- 56% more Phosphorous;
- 285% more Vitamin A;
- 208% more Vitamin B1 (Thiamine);
- 515% more Vitamin B2 (Riboflavin);
- 256% more Vitamin B3 (Niacin);

Aside from these massive increases in essential vitamins and nutrients, you also get a much higher Vitamin C content from the sprouting process. This in turn helps your body in the metabolization of proteins.

The amylase enzyme also turns a lot of the starch in grains into glucose and sucrose. Similarly, proteins are broken down into amino acids and amides. The lipase enzyme helps convert fats into fatty acids.

A visible improvement from sprouting beans instead of eating them dry is that they don't make you gassy. Plus, sprouts can help you if you're suffering from constipation due to their high fiber and water content.

You might not have known this, but - due to the high amount of vitamins and minerals - sprouts can also slow down aging. Not only that, but they also have quite a lot of male and female hormones which is easily absorbed by the body.

Want to know a sprout that's really worth growing? Try Alfalfa. Because its roots can go up to 40 feet into the ground, it can bring up some essential minerals such as manganese.

That mineral is an essential component of human insulin, so the benefit of ingesting a sprout containing it is out there. In any case, if you're not convinced by that, then how about the high content of amino acids and vitamins A, B, C, E, and K?

If you want to learn how to grow your own sprouts, then you'll find all you need to know in the following section.

Sprouting for Beginners

If you're thinking about sprouting your own food, then you're on the right track. You should obtain a nice variety of sprouting seeds for the job.

All you need to do is soak the seeds in water. First off, remember that the seeds will expand up to eight times their original size. Give them plenty of space to do so.

Make sure they are kept at an adequate temperature and that they aren't exposed to cold or intense heat. You also leave some breathing space in the container you're placing the seeds in.

Depending on the size and type of the seeds, you would keep them in water as follows:

- 5-6 hours – small seeds;
- 8 hours – medium seeds;
- 10-12 hours – beans and grains;

Then rinse, drain the water and repeat three times per day. You should see results in about two to three days. The best way to figure out when the sprouts are ready is to check for little leaves at their tips.

That is when the flavor, tenderness, and nutrients are at their peak. If you can't eat them right away, keep them in the refrigerator. They should last you about a week at most.

There are plenty of ways you can sprout seeds together. Alfalfa and broccoli come to mind. Mix in a variety of beans in a different container as well.

You can use these sprouts in many ways. Here are some examples to get you started:

- As a replacement for lettuce in salads;
- Flavoring and "beefing up" a soup;
- In sandwiches;
- To accent some of your other meals;
- Some extra vitamins in a smoothie;

If you remember, you can use sprouted almonds and nuts as nutritious snacks. Want to go one step beyond? Then sprout grains to make your own bread.

Beware the Nutrient Killers

We can't stress the importance of organically grown produce. You hear all the time about toxins and chemicals used to treat grocery store veggies and fruit. Unfortunately, that's the truth.

Think of it this way: would you consider a person who has to take 10 different medicines a day to be healthy? Sure, they may live a long life and look healthy, but their immune systems are probably crying (metaphorically speaking).

Another nutrient killer is canning. Any canned food will just lose vitamins and enzymes over time, even if you store it optimally.

Furthermore, store-bought canned items are filled to the brim with substances most people ignore. If you've ever wondered why so many people are on a diet of vegetables and pills, now you know why.

You should also know that fresh veggies and fruit start losing their nutrients the first few days after being picked. At least, if they're not kept at a proper chilly temperature or pickled.

So if you can't buy fresh from farmer markets, then get them frozen. Canned goods are best avoided.

On a final note – keep in mind what we said about steaming or blanching your food. You really want to keep those nutrients intact.

White Does not Make Right

What do sugar, white flour, salt, and homogenized dairy have in common? They've all been stripped of nutrients, and bleached to a white color to "look healthy."

In reality, white flours mostly come from GMO plants that are treated with various toxic chemicals and bleaches. This rule also applies to by-products such as white bread which is made from white flour.

The truth is that your body simply cannot process these substances. Do a little experiment: mix white flower with water and let it sit for a while. It's turned hard as a rock now. That's what you're putting inside your body.

All you're getting from white flour is spiked insulin levels and maybe constipation if you're especially lucky. "Enriched" flour doesn't mean anything – just that it was processed to be nothing like the original product.

If you can't grind your own flour, use whole-wheat or whole grain flours as a healthier alternative.

As for white sugar, it undergoes the same processes which destroy its nutrients and is grown with harmful chemicals.

In fact, it's been shown that these toxins cause cancer in sea turtles. Do you really want that kind of sugar going into your body?

A good alternative is to get sugar from health food stores. It's been pressed and dried from organically grown sugarcane, so it still preserves some nutrients.

Salt is another problem in today's diets. And we're not just talking about saltshaker salt. 85% of the salt you ingest comes from the heavily processed foods we eat daily. Avoid it as much as possible, or go for sea salt.

Our final suspect is the homogenized dairy you can find at supermarkets. That includes the hormone, steroid, and antibiotic-filled milk you buy from there.

Some of those toxins may have been left out of USDA organic milk, but it's still homogenized or pasteurized. That, in turn, destroys the nutrients we've been pressing on about, but also the enzymes you use to digest food properly.

Raw milk is the only healthy choice, but unless you know a farmer in your area that can be a problem. Don't try soy milk either, for the reasons outlined below.

Soy Is Not Really Healthy

Vegetarians will be sad to know that one of the most heavily promoted meat alternatives is not what they bargained for.

In some people, it causes thyroid issues. Foods made out of soy contain isoflavones. They block out thyroid hormone receptors, so your thyroid just can't keep up.

This, in turn, leads to increased blood sugar and eventually to increased weight on your part. But that's not even half the story. Here's what types of substances are contained in this "natural" food:

- Phytates – these prevent your gut from absorbing some essential minerals;
- Lectins;
- Oxalates;
- Protease inhibitors;
- Heavy metals (no, not the musical kind);
- Pesticide residues;

With that list, it's no wonder soy is considered one of the most allergenic foods. There is some proof that suggests soy toxins can really mess with your digestive tract, causing "leaky gut syndrome."

Larger proteins than normal are allowed into your blood stream. They can cause severe allergic reactions that naturally lead to food allergies later on.

Probably the worst soy-related incidents are the possible spikes in Type I diabetes. Type I is sometimes linked with gluten intolerance. Gluten can also pass into your bloodstream if you have a leaky gut.

Your body then produces antibodies for the foreign substance, which might end up attacking your pancreas instead.

Another after-effect of soy overconsumption is the increase in estrogen intake. Yes, soy is especially rich in estrogenic compounds. Not only that, but it could also lower testosterone levels. As such, some men report both erectile issues and increased breast size after eating soy over long periods.

Other studies point to increased chances of dementia for people who eat tofu. Gut cancers and hormone-sensitive cancers have also been linked to soy consumption.

Avoiding Soy

Unfortunately, just not eating soy-based products won't protect you from its effects. For example, if you read product labels (which you should absolutely do) you will notice soy hidden as other substances:

- Textured vegetable protein;
- Hydrolyzed plant protein;

It's also present in lots of protein-based meal replacements such as protein bars and cereals, as well as being used as a meat extender in restaurants.

Watch out for "studies" that show soy to be beneficial which are actually sponsored by corporate interests that sell soy.

For example there's a study going around that soy products prevents diabetes. How do they prove that? By assessing the phytochemical contents of a soy-based food. To the testers, the simple fact that the food contains a phytochemical is proof of its anti-diabetic properties.

The truth is much simpler than that:

- People in richer areas usually consume soy-based foods;
- Higher standards of living means better access to healthy foods;

- Lower risk of diabetes as a result;

That's all there is to it. You will never find any studies that link soy and soy-additive consumption to improved health.

What will improve it, however, are some natural fruit and veggie juices – these will be discussed below.

The Magic of Juices

If you have some cash lying around, get a juice machine. Seriously, this is the best thing you can do if you want to live a healthier lifestyle.

Why spend hundreds of dollars on supplements and take 20 of them a day to get all your vitamins? Just crush a bunch of fresh fruits and veggies with natural vitamins and minerals and get a much stronger effect.

Your body doesn't absorb artificial nutrients that well, anyway. Besides, imagine if you wanted to eat a large quantity of fruit to make up for a vitamin deficiency.

You would get sick at some point, right? Nobody can just stuff their face with fruit all day. On the other hand, if you were to drink them, perhaps all those vitamins would be easier and faster to absorb.

You can drink a glass of juice when you wake up for a boost in energy, and at night to let the nutrients work while you're sleeping.

A great hint to get all your required minerals is to include dark leafy vegetables in your drink. Spinach and cabbage are great choices.

Sure, juices don't have that much fiber content as eating the fruits raw. But the mere amount of nutrients that you absorb, and how fast you do it makes up for that fact.

As we've mentioned, fruits and veggies today are not what they once were. Every day, you pretty much have to eat 5 veggie portions and 4 portions of fruit.

Unless that's all you eat all day, it's pretty hard to do it. Not with a juicer, it isn't. Just remember to drink the juice just as you make it, as it starts to lose its nutrients soon after.

Store-bought "fresh" juices are actually pasteurized. That means those helpful enzymes and nutrients we've been talking about are gone. Plus, they contain a lot of sugars and preservatives.

Just remember to wash your produce – oh, and juice the whole thing. That's right, even the cores you generally don't eat from a fruit.

Need some juicer recommendations? Check out the Breville 800JEXL Juice Fountain Elite, or the cheaper Jack LaLane juicer.

Apple Cider Vinegar (ACV) – the Natural Diabetes Fighter

Fermented apples make up the composition of ACV. This sweet-sour liquid is full of probiotic cultures and other health benefits.

There are plenty of fine uses for ACV. Here's a quick rundown on some:

- Aiding the digestive process;
- Preventing influenza (the flu);
- Reducing inflammation;
- Balancing your pH levels;
- Relieve allergy symptoms, nausea, and heartburn;

It's a great addition to detox diets. Plus, it shows positive results in fighting some skin conditions and regulating blood sugar.

It was historically used by doctors as a treatment for many illnesses, including diabetes. There is a study made by the Nutrition Department of Arizona State University that supports this theory.

It shows that people with Type II diabetes who take two tablespoons of ACV before sleeping would lower blood sugar by up to 6% by morning.

The process is not entirely understood. It's believed to have something to do with ACV inhibiting the breakdown of starches into sugars. That, in turn, doesn't allow the body to absorb carbs as fast.

The drug Acarbose (Precose) has a similar effect. On the other hand, some believe that the vinegar just lowers blood sugar in those with high insulin resistance. This is similar to the effect of a drug called Metformin.

Natural medicines such as ACV work in synergy with the body, rather than forcing a single effect like pharmaceuticals. You're also not likely to have any side effects from ACV, as opposed to regular drugs.

Here are some of the side effects you might experience from normal medicines:

- Skin rashes;
- Weight gain and stomach issues;
- Kidney complications;
- Liver disease;
- Leg swelling;
- Dizziness, shivering, cold sweats;

Besides, apple cider vinegar can be bought for as little as two cents. Usually, diabetes medicine doesn't come alone. You have to take it in combination with some other drugs to have any effect. That could mean costs of hundreds of dollars in the long run.

A team at the Tokyo University in Japan found that ACV's acetic acid can inhibit carb-digesting enzymes from their processes. These enzymes include the following:

- Sucrose;
- Maltase;
- Lactase;
- Amylase;

When these enzymes are inhibited from doing their job of breaking down carbs, it leads to a lesser impact on your blood sugar levels. Why?

Well, the process described above allows some sugars and starches to pass through your digestive tract without being broken down.

That means your cells don't actively absorb all the sugars into your bloodstream – i.e. your blood sugar levels don't spike.

Plus, there's another great benefit to starches passing through undigested. Your gut contains beneficial bacteria that feed on all the unprocessed starches, thus aiding the digestive process.

Some studies have also shown that apple cider vinegar – when ingested – helps destroy fats. How do they do this, you might ask? Well, ACV helps "activate" some genes that break down those fats.

Many diabetics, especially those suffering from pre-diabetes and Type II diabetes, also suffer from obesity. It comes as no surprise that apple cider vinegar would bring massive benefits to those suffering from diabetes.

By the way, if you're going to take up ACV in your diet, you should know the following:

- The vinegar should be organic and unpasteurized. As we've mentioned above, pasteurization just ruins many of the benefits of otherwise healthy foods and substances;
- You can easily recognize the organic vinegar from the pasteurized vinegar by one primary trait. Namely, that ACV has a solid material that looks like a cob-web which floats around in the liquid.

That solid is actually natural cellulose. The vinegar bacteria are hard at work producing the substance when you don't destroy them through the pasteurization process.

A lot of vinegar producers today use that process. Whether they understand that they're destroying valuable nutrients and bacteria in the vinegar is a question to be discussed.

In any case, you don't have to ingest the bacterial culture in the vinegar if you don't want to. You can just use a strainer to get rid of the cellulose and other solid matter in the vinegar.

Ultimately, if you or one of your loved ones suffers from pre-diabetes or even chronic diabetes, using apple cider vinegar is a definite boon.

All they need to do is mix 1 tbsp apple cider vinegar with a glass of water and drink it. Do that three times per day about 30 minutes before eating to aid in digestion and to regulate blood sugar.

It's useful to all sorts of diabetes sufferers. Whether it's Type I, Type II, or even as a way to prevent the full-on disease for those showing symptoms of pre-diabetes

Combine its use with a natural diet consisting organic, unprocessed, unpasteurized juices and foods. The juicing processes we described in the previous sections should do wonders.

You are able to reverse the bad effects of diabetes; you just need to make some necessary changes to your diet. Don't forget to add some exercise regimens to really make things count.

PROPERLY INTERPRETING INGREDIENT LISTS

There are more than 1,500 ingredients and additives that are put into our food that are not legally required to be itemized on the ingredients list. This is something that has been made possible by the food corporations who are more interested in making money than in your health, and even government bodies that are meant to be holding our health in their highest interests. For this reason it is very important that you carefully read all of the labels on the food that you buy, because more often than not, mass-produced food is made with chemicals and other detrimental preservatives or additives. Many of these substances are not even mentioned in the ingredients list, and this applies to basically everything that you buy pre-packaged at a typical supermarket. Many companies will try to deceive you with impressive labels with promising words on them such as "natural," "fat-free," "organic," "light," "healthy," and countless others, but if it is mass-produced, it is pretty much guaranteed that those words are meaningless. The best things to look for on the label when buying food are the words "USDA organic," and it is also wise to buy locally-produced items, or those that have packaged by hand in a non-industrious environment.

DECEPTIVE FOOD LABELS

There are a number of ways that the food companies can be deceitful on their labels by printing promising words that in reality don't hold true meaning to the contents. There are many common words and characteristics that we look for when seeking out "healthy" food options, all of which come with fine print that is not mentioned on the packaging. Below are some of the most popular phrases and their real meanings:

"No Trans-Fat": If a food label claims that its contents contain zero grams of trans-fat, usually they really do contain a low number of trans-fats amounts to less than a half a gram per serving. Companies are also permitted to omit trans-fats from their labels as long as the label doesn't mention anything about fat, fatty acids, or cholesterol benefits. Even if the suggested serving size contains less than a half gram of trans-fats, generally those serving sizes are much smaller than a realistic one, so actually the trans-fats add up quickly when put in realistic quantities. As little as one gram is detrimental to your health, so this is something to be wary about when reading food labels.

"Organic": There was a ruling made in October 2005 by the Agricultural Appropriations Conference Committee that permits food items to be labeled as organic even though they may contain artificial additives, so this is another thing to be wary about. If you want real organic products, it's wisest to buy them locally.

"Low-Fat": For a version of a food product to be labeled "low-fat" or "light," the rule is that it must contain at least 25% less fat calories than the original, full-fat version of the same product. Although in some cases this may be plausible, keep in mind that a lot of the regular versions of the food products already contain enormous amounts of fat, so even the light version could hold a great deal of fat also. If you read the nutrition facts on the label, you can see for yourself how many fat calories a product has.

"Free-Range": Legally, "free-range" poultry products (including meat and eggs) are defined as the chickens being able to go outside and not forcibly confined constantly to a cage. In many cases, the minimum requirement to qualify for this is having a small opening in the chicken coop to allow the chickens to go outside for a brief period of time each day. Most of the time the chickens don't even notice this while it is available and rarely leave the coop, therefore end up spending most of their time inside of it. Consequently, "free-range" can be a rather deceitful sales ploy when the chickens are not really wandering free at all. In many cases they are also not fed a natural diet, another promise that is often made when talking about free-range products. Again, it's best to source your eggs from a vendor that you can trust gives their chickens a completely natural diet and plenty of room to roam around.

Seafood Sources: Most seafood products that you may believe to be naturally sourced or caught in the wild are actually farmed and imported from foreign countries. Farmed seafood generally holds a large amount of harmful substances, which also do not legally need to be mentioned on their packaging.

In addition to those examples listed above, the USDA also does not require foreign food producers to list harmful ingredients on their labels, but domestic producers are required to do so. However, a great majority of our food is in fact not domestically produced, including over 60% of pork products, most frozen vegetables, prepared salads (including fruit and vegetable salads), and around 95% of peanuts, pecans, and macadamia nuts. The only real standard when it comes to believing food labels is the USDA standard, but even then there are many ambiguities and things that fall through the cracks. Some words to be cautious of include "natural," "healthy," "heart-wise," and many others, since companies are able to place these words on their packaging even if the product doesn't live up to the claim.

ANALYZING THE INGREDIENTS LIST

Realistically, almost 100% of the food that you should really be consuming don't require a label at all, and are found naturally in the world with just one ingredient and without any additives. Truly organic food comes straight from nature and doesn't require any additional ingredients to be listed. It is best to buy truly organic vegetables and fruits, real free-range eggs and meat, wild meat and fish, and kosher meat, none of which should contain any added hormones, steroids, or other chemicals. Farmed seafood and meat, pasteurized dairy products, or any other food that has been contaminated with pesticides and other chemicals should be completely avoided as they are very harmful to your health. Generally speaking, when you see packaged food, you should disregard the front label and immediately refer to the ingredients list and nutrition facts. One important and basic thing that you should avoid when buying packaged food is that of sugar being listed as one of the main ingredients. This is even more true for food products that contain more than one type of sugar, including cane sugar, corn syrup, high-fructose corn syrup, dextrose, maltose, sucrose, sorbitol, xylitol, or generally anything ending with "-itol" or "-ose". Also, anything containing any amount of trans-fats (which are usually listed as hydrogenated or partially hydrogenated oils) should not be purchased at all. Also keep in mind that even if the label says there are 0 grams of trans-fats, this could be untrue due to the unrealistically stated portion sizes. If there are ANY oils listed other than coconut oil, extra virgin olive oil, or palm oil, leave it on the shelf. You should also do the same for any flour ingredients that have the words "enriched" or "refined" in front of them. It may seem like a lot of visual scouring of food labels, but if you follow these guidelines, you'll find that about 95% of foods you pick up you will place right back.

SERVING SIZES AND INGREDIENT PORTIONS

One of the most unrealistic things on every food label is the suggested serving size. When reading the nutrition facts, take note of the serving size on the label and weigh it up with how much you really eat in one portion. All of the nutrition facts and ingredients are based on the package's specified serving sizes, so if it says that a package holds four servings and you eat the whole thing, you've actually eaten quadruple the amount of everything as listed on the package. Another example is if on a packaged loaf of bread the serving size is one slice, if you eat a sandwich with two slices of bread, you have eaten double the amount of ingredients as listed on the package. Also to remember when analyzing food labels is that on the ingredients list, the order in which they are listed is based on their weight. Therefore, the first listed ingredient is the one that makes up most of the product, and the last ingredient the least.

THE HAZARDS OF GENETICALLY MODIFIED FOODS

Genetically modified organism (GMO) foods are something that you don't hear about often, but they are actually very prevalent in our food sources. While there have been some limited studies done about GMOs and their effects on certain animals (with quite alarming results), there have been no studies about the effects they can have on humans. There was one instance in particular in the late 1990s when a new kind of genetically modified corn was introduced to the food market, which contained an added gene that produces what is called BT toxin. This toxin had devastating effects on the stomachs of insects, causing them to rupture when ingested. While at the time it was said that the BT toxin is not harmful to mammals, there were some observations made that the toxin bound to the intestines of mice and Rhesus monkeys. If it can have these dreadful effects on the digestive systems in these living creatures, what effect could it have on the human body? The American Academy of Environmental Medicine believes that GMOs could cause harm to the human digestive system, in addition to a variety of other health discrepancies including allergies and autoimmune problems. Many studies done by the AAEM on GMOs' adverse effects on animals revealed an extensive list of problems caused by them, including infertility, problems with the immune system, quicker bodily aging, inconsistency in insulin levels, and problems with liver, kidney, spleen, and gastrointestinal functions. The AAEM has urged people to avoid GMO foods until further studies have been done, as there is a clear link between them and serious health problems.

The main issue with GMO foods is that they produce toxins that have never before occurred naturally, and along with it a whole plethora of health issues, and therefore we have no basis to go off of in regards to how they will effect humans in the long-term. There have been numerous instances where the consequences of introducing GMOs into the diet have been made evident, such as when GM soy was first brought into the UK. Because of the modified proteins, soy allergies in the UK grew by more than 50%. Food allergies are also growing in the US at an alarming rate, which could also possibly be a result of more GMOs in the food supply.

GMOs are actually found in many foods that we buy and eat, including artificial sweeteners, artificially sweetened beverages and food, and also corn products. In Canada, statistics showed that 93% of pregnant women, 80% of their newborn children, and nearly 70% of non-pregnant women tested positive for the BT toxin. The most common genetically modified food products available for human consumption in the United States are that of soy (94%), corn (88%), canola (90%), cottonseed (90%), and even wheat. Also pretty much anything that contains high-fructose corn syrup (which is almost anything you can buy in a typical supermarket) or is prepared using corn oil, soybean oil, cottonseed oil, or canola oil (which is commonly found in a lot of typical restaurant food) will also contain GMOs. Some other commonly GM foods are sugar beets, Hawaiian papaya, and certain kinds of zucchini and squash. Don't forget that these GM foods (such as the corn and soy) are also fed to conventionally raised and farmed animals that produce not only your meat, but also your milk, eggs, and other products. This is why it is best to buy 100% organic animal products, meaning completely grass-fed or wild-caught.

Science has proven and expressed the dangers of consuming GMOs, yet they are still prevalent in our food supply. It is calculated that approximately 30,000 items in your typical supermarket are or contain GMOs. There is also the fact that 85% of the calories that humans consume are among the most commonly GM foods, which are corn, soy, and wheat. Long story short: avoid them at all costs, since for all we know they could cause diseases that science hasn't even discovered yet.

WHAT YOUR HAIR CAN TELL YOU ABOUT YOUR BODY'S MINERALS

The way hair grows is interesting: when new cells are created, they actually absorb small amounts of the materials present in the person's bloodstream. As the new hair cells begin to emerge from the follicle, older cells get pushed out. Once this occurs, the old cells die and harden, along with all of those substances, and become your hair strands. The oil from your scalp also contains these substances, so your hair is actually the most reliable and long-term archive of what has been going through your bloodstream, more so than urine or even the blood itself. Blood and urine samples only provide what is currently going through the body, and not what has been previously within it. What's even more interesting is that depending on which area of the strand is analyzed (how far down the length or close to the scalp), you can see how much of which substances were present during a certain time period. Besides being able to tell what is or has been inside the bloodstream, it can also tell what has not been there, such as essential vitamins and minerals. Vitamin deficiencies as well as excesses can be examined through hair analysis, and therefore point to or give explanation to any medical issues a person may be experiencing. For example, if your hair reveals an excess of calcium in the body, that could lead to arteriosclerosis, which is the hardening of the arteries as a result of a buildup of calcium plaque. Conversely, a deficiency of calcium in the body can lead to osteoporosis and make a person more prone to bone fractures, teeth issues, muscle cramps, and a variety of other issues.

THE IMPORTANCE OF TESTING MINERAL LEVELS

Analyzing the hair strands can uncover many different mineral deficiencies and disparities in the body that can cause many metabolic discrepancies, even before symptoms arise. Minerals and vitamins are an essential component in the body's functions, and take part in almost all of the body's enzyme processes, without which we could not survive. Hair analysis is a great tool to prevent serious issues before they get too far. It is especially useful in patients who are experiencing health problems either with no explanation, or if ineffective treatment is pointing towards an incorrect diagnosis. Aside from more serious problems, vitamin and mineral deficiencies (often caused by a poor diet) can lead to small abnormalities or changes in the body, including:

- White spots in fingernails, caused by a zinc deficiency
- Vertical ridges in nails, caused by an iron deficiency
- Weak or easily breakable hair and nails, caused by a disproportion in copper and calcium
- Deep indentations across nails, caused by a calcium deficiency
- Stretch marks, caused by a zinc deficiency
- Stunted growth, caused by a zinc deficiency

- Mood swings, arthritis, and chronic pain and fatigue, possibly caused by a buildup of toxic metals in the body such as lead, mercury, cadmium, or aluminum
- Pre-menstrual headaches, caused by an excess of copper in the system
- Exacerbated infections, caused by an overly excessive intake of Vitamin C
- Adolescent acne, caused by a zinc deficiency and/or copper or lead poisoning

The most common reason for having mineral deficiencies or disparities is that of a poor diet, often including consuming too many refined carbohydrates and sugars. Some specific diets can cause mineral imbalances as well, such as strict vegetarian and vegan diets, or other ones that are based off of leaving out a particular food group. Improper diets are capable of causing more severe and long-term health problems also, such as constipation, diverticulitis, and heart disease. Taking vitamin supplements that may not be well-suited for an individual's body is also a cause of imbalances. Some other factors that can influence mineral and vitamin concentration or lack thereof in the body include certain medications (including contraceptive pills), stress, work factors, heredity, and environmental issues. Approximately 80% of the population suffers from mineral and vitamin deficiencies that inhibit enzyme reactions and also negatively affect stomach acid which can detriment the digestive system. Analyzing the hair strands is the most efficient way to observe an individual's blood makeup and determine what minerals are missing or that they have too much of.

There are countless other conditions and problems that can arise from vitamin and mineral discrepancies. Too much lead in the system can cause hyperactivity in children as well as multiple sclerosis, and mercury toxicity in a pregnant mother can cause in-utero death of a child. Blood sugar inconsistencies are a common cause of obesity, and zinc deficiencies can inhibit potency in men as a result of the prostate not having enough of it. A lack of zinc in the system can also stunt bone growth and prevent the proper development of sex organs, as well as cause blood sugar imbalances. Brain damage in alcoholics can be caused by magnesium deficiencies. Medications such as diuretics (generally given to patients with heart and kidney problems) can cause a potassium deficiency. Too much copper and iron can contribute to migraine headaches and even schizophrenia. More serious illnesses and conditions caused by vitamin and mineral discrepancies as well as metal toxicities are heart problems, diabetes, a variety of mental disorders, feminine conditions, epilepsy, kidney disease, anemia, leukemia, and other types of cancers.

It's important to keep in mind that doctors often misdiagnose conditions. They may say you have a certain illness that could possibly simply be a vitamin or mineral issue and prescribe unnecessary medication for it. While the medication may relieve some of the symptoms, the underlying problem can still exist and continue to cause damage. Hair analysis can quickly determine many of these

problems and rule out more serious illnesses that you
otherwise may be falsely diagnosed with.

TESTING YOUR OWN BLOOD SUGAR AND KEEPING DIABETES OFF THE RECORD

Being formally diagnosed with diabetes can be
disadvantageous for your insurance rates—it can either
make your current rates skyrocket, or may even completely
prevent you from being able to get health or life insurance
at all. If you're worried this may happen to you if you go to
the doctor to get tested, it is possible to test your own blood
sugar at home by yourself and avoid the risk of diabetes
being placed on your medical records. You can buy
inexpensive self-testing kits at a number of stores without a
referral from you doctor and test both your post-meal and
fasting blood sugar levels yourself at home. If you already
have been officially diagnosed with diabetes or prediabetes, there's still a solution. With the self-testing kits as
well as the information you'll find in this book, you can
make changes yourself to help regulate your blood sugar
levels. When you return to your doctor for follow-up
testing, they can then state on your files that you are no
longer diabetic or pre-diabetic.

To get started, first purchase a low-priced meter and test
strips at a drug store, supermarket, online, or at some other
stores like Wal-Mart or Target. Meters generally come with
test strips, lancets, and a lancing device included, but if not,
go ahead and buy a small package. Note that test strips
usually expire three months after opening the box, so don't

purchase more than about ten strips for a single person. If you like, you can also buy further tests to see how your body responds to certain kinds of foods. Every meter operates differently, so make sure to read the instructions. It's best to do a few practice runs before doing your first actual test. It is extremely important to note that reusing a lancet multiple times is fine if only testing one person's blood levels, but you must NEVER use the same lancet for two different people. If you notice that pricking your finger hurts a little more than usual after a few times, then your lancet is probably getting dull and will need to be changed.

Another thing to note is that in a hospital setting, blood sugar levels are tested as "plasma glucose," of which the resulting glucose measurements are usually about 10-12% higher than that of a "whole blood-based" test. While most of the self-testing kits are also for plasma glucose, some are also meant for whole blood. Check which one applies to your own testing kit, and if it is for whole blood, just add the 10-12% for results more similar to that of a professional lab. One good self-testing kit is the "TRUE result" blood glucose starter kit, which costs only $5.94 including shipping from Amazon.com, which includes the meter itself, ten test strips, ten lancets, a lancing device, logbook, instruction booklet, and a carrying case.

It's best to do your first test of the day first thing in the morning after waking up, and before eating or drinking anything. Make sure your hands are clean with warm water and soap, and lance one of your fingertips; many people find that using the side of your finger instead of the pad is less painful. Also, the littlest finger tends to produce the most blood, but of course, you can experiment and see what works the best for you. Start off with the most shallow setting on your lancet (generally this will be labeled as setting "1"), and if it isn't deep enough to draw enough blood, put it up one notch at a time until it works. Also it is not recommended to first dab your finger with rubbing alcohol or another disinfectant prior to lancing, seeing as this can dry the skin out and make it more difficult to draw blood. Test the blood sugar with the meter and then write down the result. This is what is called your "fasting blood sugar." If the reading is surprisingly high, wash your hands again and retest. Even if you have a small amount of sugar on the place where you lance it, it can drastically skew the results.

As stated previously, it is absolutely necessary that each separate person uses a different lancet and that they are never shared. This is to prevent the transmission of any blood-borne illnesses, even if they may be unknown. For a single person, it is not necessary to use a fresh lancet for each test. People report to change their lancets about once a month, or sometimes even less often. Just remember that if a lancing device is being shared between two or more people, you MUST change the lancets between uses!

When throwing away your used test strips, it's good to know that blood products are classified as medical waste. If you don't have access to an official bio-waste bin, you can simply use an old detergent bottle. Once it is full, seal the top shut and label it with "Caution: Medical Waste." Look up what your local trash disposal regulations are and act accordingly. You can buy some affordable bio-waste and sharps disposal containers online, such as from Amazon.com.

After your initial morning test, you should test again right after a meal, preferably something that contains 60-70 grams of fast-acting carbohydrates. A large bagel is a good food for this, but if you are gluten-free, you can also eat a large boiled potato or a cup of cooked white rice. Make sure, however, not to add fats to this meal such as butter, cheese, peanut butter, or other similar toppings, since they can slow down the carbohydrate digestion process. As you begin eating, write down the time, and set three alarms for one, two, and three hours later. When your first timer goes off, go ahead and wash your hands (or use an alcohol pad or hand sanitizer if you don't have access to soap and water) and test your blood sugar again, also writing down the results. Repeat the process for the second and third timers. After this, your testing is done and you can continue with your regular meals for the day.

One thing to note if you are on a low-carb diet (usually less than 75 grams of carbohydrates per day) is that testing after a meal will generally give you slightly higher results than if eating a diet that consists of over 150 grams of carbohydrates per day. If a post-meal glucose tolerance test is requested by a doctor, a person must eat 150 grams of carbohydrates for three days prior to having the test done in order to get the most accurate results. However, if you would like to do this at home and do not wish to deviate from your low-carb diet, there is another calculation that you can do to adjust your results accordingly. A low-carb diet provisionally elevates post-meal glucose values, especially if a person eats a large amount of carbohydrates that they are not used to eating. To calculate for the difference, subtract 10 mg/dl from any test results following a meal after two hours that is over 140 mg/dl. It is not an exact calculation, but is accurate enough for home tests.

Deciphering Your Test Results and Accounting for the Meter's Margin of Error

As you would probably gather, home tests tend to be slightly less accurate than a professional lab test done in a hospital. However, there are two ways to work around this. You can either purchase a calibrating solution for your meter (which can also be easily purchased online) to determine the exact margin of error compared to that of a lab test, or you can simply account for a +/- 5% difference.

As stated previously, there is a slight difference between the calculations of "plasma glucose" and "whole blood" when testing blood sugar levels. All of the meters currently available in the USA are based on plasma glucose calculations, but in some other countries such as the UK, many meters are still based on whole blood calculations. The blood sugar testing topics discussed in this book will be in regards to plasma glucose levels, so if you are using a whole blood meter, simply multiply the results by 1.2 to reach the plasma glucose measurements.

An ideal blood sugar is a result that is below 100 mg/dl after all of the post-meal tests. If you have gotten this result, you do not need to do any further testing and can continue as you were. The average blood sugar levels are below 140 mg/dl after one hour of eating the carbohydrates and below 120 mg/dl after two hours. According to the Joslin Diabetes Clinic of Harvard Medical School, this is the maximum level to be considered as having a normal level.

For results at the upper end of the normal range (so around 140 mg/dl after one hour and 120 mg/dl after two hours), there could be either beta cell dysfunction or insulin resistance present. If this describes your results, especially if it comes along with weight gain, a good solution is to lower the amount of carbohydrates ingested daily and combine it with a good exercise program. If your blood sugar results are above 140 mg/dl after one hour or above 120 mg/dl after two hours, this qualifies as pre-diabetes in accordance with the American Diabetes Association. Doctors also refer to this as impaired glucose tolerance, or IGT.

If your results are pointing to pre-diabetes, it is very important that you take action and don't let it sit. With the extra glucose molecules in your body, they will eventually bond to proteins in your body and insert themselves into the arteries, cause kidney damage, obstruct retinal capillaries, decrease nerve function, and cause impotency and pain. If you allow this to continue, within a few years it will develop into full-blown diabetes, which generally entails permanent damage. The good news is that if you catch it early, there is a chance for you to eradicate the pre-diabetes factors through weight loss, decreasing carbohydrate intake, and exercising more. Keeping up this routine can ensure that your blood sugar returns to and remains at a normal level. If you notice your results may be pointing to pre-diabetes, talk about it with your doctor. If they seem nonchalant about it, seek a second opinion immediately.

It is important to act as soon as possible after seeing an abnormal result in your blood sugar levels. If you wait too long and your fasting blood sugar reaches a level of 126 mg/dl, this is the level at which doctors generally consider diabetic. At this point, there is a chance that a minimum of half of the pancreatic beta cells could be dead and unable to renew. If at any time during testing your blood sugar levels rose above 200 mg/dl, it is vital that you see a doctor as soon as possible, as this qualifies as a diabetes diagnoses according to the American Diabetes Association.

Aside from elevated blood sugar levels, another problem is not having your levels high enough, which is referred to as hypoglycemia. If your blood sugar fluctuates after the two- and three-hour tests and at any point drops below 70 mg/dl, this is called "reactive hypoglycemia". What occurs in this case is that after ingesting carbohydrates, the blood sugar rises, but the body releases too much insulin to bring the blood sugar back down. This can also lead to an eventual diabetes diagnosis, although it can take up to ten years before it is noticed. Aside from being at risk for diabetes, hypoglycemia can also point to insulin resistance, which causes an increase of insulin production that drastically lowers the blood sugar. This can eventually lead to heart disease, so it is also vital to talk about this with a healthcare professional. Eating a diet that is high in protein and low in carbohydrates can prove effective in managing hypoglycemia.

If you have any unusual blood sugar levels following post-meal tests, it is wise to ask your doctor to perform an annual HbA1c test. As the official diabetes levels as described by the lab standards tend to be way higher than a harmful level, take note of the results yourself and keep track of whether it remains consistent or is increasing. If your results at any point rise above 5.7%, which is the level at which doctors normally say you are at risk for diabetes, you need to start really taking your blood sugar levels into your own hands. It is very doable to regulate your own blood sugar levels by cutting out fast-acting carbs, such as those found in soft drinks, candy, white flour, potatoes, and white rice. As stated previously, the idea of the perfect blood sugar level is that of 100 mg/dl or less after one hour of eating, and then to remain at a steady level of between 70-90 mg/dl. Keep in mind that the lower your blood sugar levels are after eating, the less chance you have of developing diabetes or heart disease. Also an important thing to do is make sure you are getting enough sleep every night so that your body can revitalize itself regularly.

A Diabetes Diet That's Worth It

A "diabetes diet" probably sounds better to you than a "weight loss diet." That's because it actually is!

Everybody's motivation sinks when they hear they need to control their weight to deal with diabetes. But this time it's serious. When your life is at risk, there's no turning back from dieting.

You've probably heard, or even know people with Type 2 diabetes. For half their lives they try to diet their way to a healthier weight and lifestyle.

Not all of them succeed, however. In fact, without strong willpower, it might seem impossible to some.

Of course it seems that way when your mind keeps telling you the only way to health is through intense dieting. Rest assured in the fact that a diabetes diet doesn't mean you have to starve yourself to lose weight.

On the contrary, the purpose of such a diet is to regulate your blood sugar levels so they stop being life-threatening. You know what that means, right?

You can eat as much as you want, but you need to be careful what you eat. Some foods increase your blood sugar, and that's the last thing you want to do.

The weight loss is just a bonus from this diet, not a means to an end. Here are the aspects that contribute to your weight loss from a diabetes diet:

- When your body produces too much blood sugar, it needs to produce more insulin as well;
- That means your body becomes resistant to insulin;
- In effect, your cells absorb much more glucose than needed, causing the leftover glucose to become fat.

Lower your blood sugar, and that doesn't happen anymore. It also contributes to quelling the feeling of hunger you get from fluctuating blood sugar levels.

That's right; you can finally stop your hunger pangs with a well-suited diet. How? Just read on.

Carbohydrate Control is the Key

You will need a blood sugar meter for these next steps towards a healthier life. This may sound tedious in writing, but it doesn't actually take up much time.

Measure your blood sugar. You will need to do this one, two, and three hours after every meal. Check that your blood sugar does not pass the following values:

- 1 hour – 140 mg/dl
- 2 hours – 120 mg/dl
- 3 hours – 100 mg/dl

Foods rich in carbohydrates are more likely to give you those dangerously high values. All you need to do now is avoid those foods. That's all there is to it!

Yes, you will have to sacrifice some of your favorite dishes. Just remember all the goodies you still get to eat, and everything will be just fine.

Now, you might be thinking: "Are fats a major contributor to my predicament?" The truth is that carbohydrates are the usual suspect you should watch out for.

Eating fatty foods on the regular is probably not a good idea – but it is carbohydrates that form triglycerides that you should be worried about.

Otherwise, your diet will not suffer from any extra proteins or fats you ingest. And speaking of suffering, you should probably start easing the job of your beta cells (the ones that make insulin).

More info below.

Helping Out Your Beta Cells

Now, the information above will help you reduce your blood sugar after meals. But what if you have increased levels even when you're fasting?

Obviously, a diet low in carbs will aid your pancreas somewhat. Unfortunately, there's only so much it can do without the assistance of its compromised beta cells.

So what can you do? Well, before you head to sleep, you can have a light snack. It might seem counter-productive when you're trying to diet. But remember what we said in the beginning? You're not doing it to lose weight.

As such, a protein bar works wonders. According to Marion J. Franz, MS, RD, LD, "50–60% of protein becomes glucose and enters the bloodstream about 3–4 hours after it's eaten."

A couple of crackers work just as well. Just remember to test their effects on your blood sugar. That's how you know if they work for your condition.

Many people don't like being told what they can, and cannot eat. Doesn't it feel better knowing that you decide what's best based on your own experiences?

A Helpful Checklist

We've gone over this information already, but to make it easier for you, we'll create a checklist that's easy to follow:

- Start a food diary (a spreadsheet works best) – write down everything you eat. As more items show up on your list, you will run out of foods to test out, and you can just consider past results.
- Remember to test your blood sugar. Do it just after you've woken up, and right before a meal (so you can compare results).
- Test your sugar again as described initially: one, two, and three hours after you've eaten. You can also test it after four hours if the values aren't back to normal by then.
- Write everything down in your spreadsheet.

Soon enough, you will get used to this schedule, and you will have found out what food you should avoid. The following section will discuss some examples that will give you a higher reading.

What Causes Blood Sugar to Skyrocket?

Bread, fruit, starches, sugars, cereals, potatoes, wheat by-products. These are the likely suspects that will do damage.

Do test them out, though. It differs from case to case. If you find that some of those increase your blood sugar, at least you've crossed them off your list.

Replace the lost carbs from those food items with vegetables instead. They should help you get back to normal levels.

What are those levels? Well, aside from those we presented initially, a non-diabetic person would get the following readings:

- Between 70 mg/dl and 90 mg/dl without having eaten – this is the ideal.
- Under 100 mg/dl – not healthy, but acceptable levels.

As long as your blood sugar doesn't hit 140 mg/dl two hours after a meal, you should be safe. Of course, that's an extreme case. You should always strive for better numbers!

The reason is that those readings can tell you a lot about any problems that might arise in time. For example, if you don't keep your blood sugar levels in check you might end up with heart complications.

Everybody's body chemistry is different. This is why no one diet will fit every lifestyle. We've tried to allow you as much freedom as possible.

For example, some people might not tolerate wheat or rice-based products but have no problem with corn.

Similarly, they might not stand the sugar in honey or canned fruit. On the other hand, the sugar in fresh fruits such as watermelons would cause no issues.

In the end, it's much better if you understand how your body works than if somebody just hammers a fad diet into your head. Learning and exploration can also help you keep on track.

It's also not uncommon to find people who keep eating the same things over and over. This is a chance for you to explore and experiment with different recipes as well.

Ultimately, this is how you benefit from creating your own diabetes diet:

- You will finally have normal blood sugar levels;
- You can avoid insulin injections and medicine which can have adverse effects;
- The best of all? No horrible end results such as blindness, strokes, or even amputations;

Begin your diet today, feel the effects starting tomorrow!

What to Substitute When You Are Cutting Carbs

We all know that those people who follow a healthy, well-balanced meal plan reduce their risk of getting chronic ailments. Diabetes is mostly the result of unhealthy eating habits. Reducing your carbohydrate intake can help control blood sugar as well as encourage weight loss and increased energy.

Here are a few useful food suggestions to get you started on the road to fitness.

Lower your blood sugar by reducing the amount of carbs you consume. Monitor you serving sizes. Portion control helps regulate calorie intake and subsequent blood sugar spikes. It can also lead to weight loss. Stick to fruits, vegetables, whole grains and unsaturated fats. There are many nutritious oils that can be used instead of unhealthy fats, so avoid these at all costs.

Fill up on fiber-rich food. This helps to prevent overeating and slows carb digestion and sugar absorption while promoting a more gradual rise in blood sugar levels.

Drinking enough water will help you keep your blood sugar levels within healthy limits. In addition to preventing dehydration, water helps your kidneys flush out excess blood sugar.

Your health can be largely improved by making just a few simple changes in your eating habits. If you're afraid such changes in your diet will cost an arm and a leg, this couldn't be further from the truth. It is possible to eat healthy on a budget. You just have to be aware of what you eat.

Once you decide on a low carb plan, stick to it. Broaden your culinary horizons and be adventurous in the kitchen. If your meals are boring, you will soon be bored with the diet.

Shop smart and look for bargains. Plan and prepare meals. And don't waste those leftovers. They can create quick, delicious meals.

Portions of low carb veggies are a must with all your meals. Capsicums, broccoli, asparagus, mushrooms, zucchini, spinach, avocados, cauliflower, green beans, cucumbers, lettuce, and cabbage - there's a wide range of healthy low carb greens to choose from, so go for it. They can only do you good! Some veggies have a high carb content so eat these in small amounts. In general, veggies growing above ground are low carb and can be eaten freely. Vegetables growing below ground contain more carbs, so you have to be more careful of them.

Eating foods rich in chromium and magnesium help prevent deficiencies and reduce blood sugar problems. Chromium-rich foods include egg yolks, whole grain products, high-bran cereals, coffee, nuts, green beans, broccoli, and meat. Magnesium-rich foods include dark leafy greens, whole grains, fish, dark chocolate, bananas, avocados, and beans.

Breakfast is the most important meal of the day and yet so many people skip it. Basis eggs and meat breakfasts are low carb meals that will produce improved blood sugar results since most people have a higher resistance to insulin in the morning. Just add boiling water to ground flax meal. Add a scoop of whey protein powder and flavor with a sprinkling of nuts or grated coconut. Delicious, and such a good start for your day! Who doesn't love pancakes? Make them with whey protein powder and top them up with low carb fresh or frozen fruit. Raspberries, or strawberries, or any berries for that matter, work perfectly for this low carb energy breakfast.

Lunch can be as interesting as you make it. You can find plenty of low carb meal plans online to suit your palate and budget. Steam or boil cauliflower and puree it. A dash of cream, butter and salt, and you have a yummy substitute for those mashed potatoes that you have to stay away from. Cabbage and lettuce leaves make great wraps so long as your filler is low carb. You will have to give up pasta, but strips of steamed carrots, cucumbers, eggplant, or zucchini topped with your favorite sauce will hit the spot. The same goes for pizza. Order one and just eat the topping. Or use crust free recipes. They're delicious and easy to prepare at home.

No need to give up rolls, though. Add them to your meal plan if you can eat gluten. Choose a low carb recipe and make a whole batch. Save them in a plastic container and keep them in the freezer. They're so handy when you need a low carb snack.

Don't be afraid of snacking. There are plenty of low carb, quality fat, and high protein choices to satisfy those munchies. Imaginative meal planning will create amazing substitutes and leave no place for carb cravings. Find out how to use low calorie, low carb foods as a healthy snack to get you through between meal hunger pangs. Crisply baked fine slices of cheese or veggies make ideal snacks. Sprinkle dried cranberries and toasted slivers of almonds over a cup of plain yogurt. Or get a good dose of fiber by mixing unsweetened miniature shredded wheat with dried cranberries and a tablespoon of roasted almonds and pistachios.

Nuts are a healthy addition to your low carb diet but make sure you check their food values. Some can be really high in calories and carbs. In reasonable quantities, almonds, walnuts, pecans, sunflower seeds, and pumpkin seeds are low carb and full of healthy oils that lower cholesterol. Eat them raw for best nutritional value as cooking destroys the natural digestive enzymes and natural vitamins.

Eating out doesn't have to scuttle the low carb diet plan. Make smart choices by avoiding the sugars, starches, and fried food options on the menu. These items may taste good but they will do your body harm. And watch out for the dressings. The ingredients used in most restaurants will likely cause damaging sugar spikes. Better to choose places that have healthy menu selections. You can't go wrong with steak, chicken, salads, or sea food, grilled, toasted or steamed. You can enjoy guilt free, low carb, nutritious meals when dining out too.

Stay away from sugar, HFCS, wheat, seed oils, trans-fats, 'diet' and 'low-fat' products and highly processed foods. Read the fine print on labels. Watch out for erroneous advertising that passes off 'low carb' foods that are actually high carb and full of toxic additives. These contain ingredients that raise blood sugar. Some will turn into blood glucose as soon as it hits your digestive tract.

Be sure to check with your doctor before making healthy low carb meal changes. This is particularly important if you have problems with blood sugar control or if you are taking medications to lower your sugar levels. But do start doing something about cutting carbs for a healthier lifestyle. It's really quite simple and the results are so worth it.

Sugars are harmful for the body

Sugars come in many forms beside the white granules we use. Corn syrup, honey, and maple syrup are all sugars. We now consume sugars in large amounts. The human body is not able to cope with this massive intake of refined carbs and as a result our vital organs are severely damaged. Refined sugar is a dangerous food which is extremely harmful for the body. It is pure energy without any essential nutrients and therefore should be avoided completely. The consumption of sugars is the main cause of many ailments including obesity, and heart and liver disease. Sugary foods nourish bacteria in the mouth and cause erratic spikes in blood sugar levels. This can produce mood swings, fatigue, and headaches. Sugars creates insulin resistance which leads to metabolic syndrome and diabetes. Artificial sweeteners are as unhealthy as refined sugar and significantly increase the risk for a number of health problems. It is better to keep sugars away from ones food since they contribute nothing but harm for the body.

Health benefits of fats

Not all fats are the same and some can be beneficial for your health. Even though they have a higher calorie count than carbs or proteins, there are 'good' fats that can lower blood cholesterol levels, decrease the risk of heart disease, and stabilize insulin and blood sugar. Bad fats, on the other hand, can cause obesity and increase the risk of certain diseases. It's important to know the difference between good fats and bad fats. Healthy fats from fish, avocados, olives, nuts, and seeds are beneficial for your brain and mood. Good fats are vital for your physical and emotional health. Avoid bad fats found in commercially baked bread, cakes, and cookies. Packaged foods such as popcorn, chips, and candy, have bad fats as do fried foods and many cooking oils. Use natural olive or coconut oil and make sure you discard anything with 'hydrogenated' in its ingredients.

Water is vital for survival

Most of the earth's surface is made up of water. The adult human body is sixty percent water. Our planet couldn't function without water. It effects the climate and determines tides. Plants, animals, and human beings could not survive without water. The billions of cells in our bodies must have water to live. If you ignore the opportunity to hydrate the cells, they start dying at an abnormal rate. This large number of dehydrated dead cells clog up the circulatory system, kidneys and liver. Replacing new cells cannot be done normally in a body cluttered with dead cell toxins. Full functioning is impossible without the necessary cells.

Water is part of all our body functions and processes. It carries nutrients around the body and in the blood, helps chemical reactions to take place, replaces the loss of fluids, and gets rid of waste products. Water is consumed by drinking and absorbed by the skin when we bathe or swim. It provides oxygen to the brain, increases our metabolic rate, helps the body burn fat, and keeps us alert and active. Lack of water consumption creates dehydration which causes fatigue, and in extreme cases, even death. Drinking enough water daily balances the lymph system which helps you perform your daily functions, balance your body fluids, and fight infection. This treatment cleanses the colon and enables the body to absorb nutrients from food. It increases the production of new blood cells and helps with weight loss. Water helps to purges the toxins from the blood and as a result, your skin will be clear and glowing.

Water the human body regularly

The human body must consume water daily, many times a day. It is a vital part of health, nutrition, and quality life. The recommended amount of water to drink within twenty-four hours is 2 liters or 8 eight ounce glasses. The general rule is to divide your body weight by two and that the amount of water ounces should be taken in twenty-four hours. This does not include other fluids you drink. More or less may be consumed depending on the climate, body weight, and activity levels. We lose water from our bodies mainly through sweat and urine. Urine should be clear if you drink enough water. If it is yellow, it means you are not drinking enough and this will affect the elimination of body wastes, so increase your intake.

Remember, drinking juices, tea, coffee, or alcohol does not count in your daily water intake. Alcohol actually dehydrates the body so addition water must be consumed to make up the loss of fluids. Dehydration can also be due to exercise or heat and this condition will effect physical and mental performance. Certain medications could cause a dry mouth. Increased thirst can be caused by untreated diabetes. Some circumstances do require an increased intake of water. Overhydrating, or drinking too much water can unbalance the water and sodium in the body and have dangerous consequences so see what works for you within the recommended intake range.

Try the amazing water cure

Many people do not drink as much water as they should. This does not allow the body to do its job to get rid of all the impurities that collect inside us. Being aware of this can change lazy habits and induce us to reach for regular drinks of pure water throughout the day. This should become a lifetime habit and not just a fad for a few days. Keeping your body hydrated may be all it takes to bring back your health and energy. It may even cure some of those ailments that have been bothering you. Drinking water in the morning as soon as you wake up is known to have amazing therapeutic effects on a whole list of health conditions including headaches, pain, asthma, and cancer. Try drinking half your body weight in ounces of pure water each day if you want the best results.

The best time to have a drink of water is in the morning on an empty stomach because it hydrates the cells of all the organs and the blood supply. Having that morning drink of water before you brush your teeth cleanses your system. If we eat breakfast without watering our cellular system we begin killing our cells. The remains of this dead matter piles up and the body becomes a dump for toxins. This will impair the body's functioning and lead to disease and organ failure. Try to avoid all liquids half an hour before and after meals. You may have a few sips of water during meals if you must but remember, drinking water dilutes the acids in the stomach that are needed to digest food. Dehydration is the cause of many of our disorders so keep a bottle of water with you at all times. You will have a ready supply on hand and be able to take sips of water regularly throughout the day. Having a drink of water is the best tonic and costs nothing. There's no better deal than that!

EFFECTS OF ALCOHOL ON DIABETES

If you have diabetes and plan on drinking alcohol, there are three questions that you should ask yourself as suggested by the American Diabetes Association. The first thing to consider is if your diabetes is under control. Secondly, you should consult with your doctor and make sure that you don't have any other health issues that could be exacerbated by alcohol, such as nerve damage or high blood pressure. Lastly, you need to make sure you are educated on the effects that alcohol can have on you if you are living with diabetes.

Alcohol is metabolized by the liver instead of the stomach, and each drink takes approximately two hours to be fully metabolized. Even though this is true, within five minutes of drinking an alcoholic beverage, there is enough alcohol in your bloodstream to be measured. If you drink alcohol at a rate faster than it can be metabolized by your liver, this is what causes that familiar "buzz" or drunkenness, with the extra alcohol moving to different parts of your body, most notably your brain. Alcohol in combination with many diabetic medications or supplements such as insulin, sulfonylurea (glipizide, glyburide), and meglitinide

(Prandin) can cause your blood sugar to drop hazardously low, since your liver switches its focus over to filtering the alcohol out of your blood rather than stabilizing your blood sugar. Therefore, it is best to completely avoid alcohol if you have low blood glucose, but if you do drink, it is imperative not to do so on an empty stomach, since food slows down the absorption rate of alcohol into the bloodstream. Immediately upon drinking an alcoholic beverage and for up to twelve hours thereafter, you are at risk for hypoglycemia. If you do plan on drinking, make sure to carry your test kit with you to make sure your glucose levels are safe, and also keep on hand glucose tablets or other forms of sugar. Keep in mind that in the case of alcohol consumption, Glucagon shots will not help you. According to the American Diabetes Association, regardless of if a person is diabetic or not, the recommended amount of alcohol consumption per day is one drink for women and two drinks for men. Binge drinking can be especially dangerous, given the fact that drunkenness and hypoglycemia have similar symptoms, including dizziness, disorientation, and sleepiness. It is advisable to wear a medical ID if you have diabetes, especially if you plan on drinking, since making a mistake between identifying hypoglycemia and drunkenness can be a devastating error.

FOODS THAT BURN FAT AND HELP YOU LOSE WEIGHT

Protein is an entire food group with a variety of different foods that are great for aiding in fat and weight loss. Since all proteins are thermogenic, they require that your body to uses more energy and time in order to digest them. Protein takes a great deal longer to digest than fats and carbs, with as much as 30% of calories that you ingest from protein being used just for digestion. Conversely, fat and carbs use only 2% of sugar calories for digestion and are either used immediately for energy, and if the body's activity level is too low to warrant its direct use (which is often the case), it is stored as excess fat, and even more leaves you hungry sooner. Protein, on the other hand, leaves you with a full feeling for a longer amount of time, and 30% of the calories are burned off for the digestion process, meaning much less calories will be stored as fat as opposed to those of fat and carbs.

Oatmeal is a great food to start the day with, as it also keeps you full for a decent amount of time and therefore limits the amount of calories you are likely to take in at one time. Besides this, it also provides you with long-lasting energy. Oatmeal is very fiber-rich and regulates your insulin levels, which is a key component to fat loss. The reason for this is that insulin facilitates fat storage, especially if you are not very physically active. For a healthy breakfast, have a bowl of oatmeal (not the pre-mixed sweetened packages) or baby cereal, along with raw milk, almond milk, rice milk, or kefir, with some added stevia if you like a bit of sweetness. You should really aim to avoid soy milk. You can add on the side a couple of scrambled or poached eggs, and drink a cup of Rooibos herbal tea or fresh fruit and/or vegetable juice.

Drinking cold water also has a small yet effective influence. Everyone knows that drinking water is one of, if not the, most vital components of any diet, but drinking it cold can have an even better effect on managing your weight. It has been shown that drinking cold water requires more calories to warm it up before it can go through your stomach, thus increasing your metabolism. The other numerous benefits include keeping your body hydrated, which better enables absorption of energy and encouraging fat loss. Drinking water and keeping your body hydrated also in general tends to reduce your calorie intake. It is best to drink some cold water as soon as you wake up, as well as up to a half hour before eating any food. To determine how much water you should be drinking daily, divide your body weight in half and convert it into ounces, and this is how much water you should be drinking per day. This amount does not account for any other kinds of beverages.

Eggs are one protein in particular that is especially beneficial to your health and can contribute to weight loss. Instead of having carbs for breakfast such as bagels or toast, eating two eggs keeps you full for a longer period of time and can decrease your overall calorie consumption for up to 24 hours. Eggs have an abundant amino acid profile, which make them a great aid in building muscles. Building up lean muscle while weight training is a good contribution to your health, because it causes your body to constantly burn calories. You may hear that the yolk is actually much less beneficial than the white, but this is quite untrue. Egg yolks are the most healthy and vitamin-rich part of the egg, also with healthy fats that inhibit hunger and encourage slow digestion. The yolk of the egg consist of over 90% of its calcium, iron, phosphorous, zinc, thiamin, vitamin B6, folate, vitamin B12, and pantothenic acid. Not only that, but the egg yolks also hold all of its fat-soluble vitamins (A, D, E, and K), in addition to all of its essential fatty acids. Whole eggs are also more beneficial than eating just the egg whites because the whites contain considerably less micronutrients than that of the yolks, and the yolks help construct a stable amino acid profile. It is also advised to buy free-range organic eggs from chickens that have been fed a natural, nutrient-rich diet, which regulates the beneficial omega-3 fatty acids and inflammatory omega-6 fatty acids.

Specific oils that contain healthy fats are also vital for a healthy, functioning body. Oils containing healthy fats include coconut oil, palm oil, macadamia oil, and extra virgin olive oil. These kinds of fats encourage the action of uncoupling proteins, which are chemicals that signal the body to burn extra calories instead of storing them. A good way to incorporate these oils into your diet is to include a tablespoon to your protein shakes, or combine with balsamic vinegar to make a low-fat and low-carb salad dressing.

Avocados are also a great source of healthy fats. In addition to being full of monounsaturated fat, avocados are also rich in vitamins, minerals, micronutrients, antioxidants, and fiber. Avocados are a delicious component of any diet and can be prepared in a variety of ways, the most popular being in the form of guacamole. You can either make it at home or buy it pre-made at the store, but just make sure to read the label if you buy store-bought guacamole to make sure that it contains no added sugars, creams, or unhealthy oils such as soybean or canola oil. It is best to have entirely natural and vegetable-based guacamole, such as garlic, tomatoes, onions, and seasonings. You can also eat plain sliced avocados on sandwiches, burgers, salads, and a variety of egg dishes. The healthy fats and nutrients in avocados assist in stabilizing hormones that encourage fat loss and the building up of muscles. Also, avocados are another one of those foods that keeps you full for a long period of time after eating them.

Another group of food that contains healthy fats that assist in fat-burning are nuts and legumes, including walnuts, almonds, pecans, macadamia nuts, and many others. Although the nuts themselves do consist primarily of fat (between 75-90%), similarly to avocados, this is all healthy fat. They also contain many vitamins, minerals, antioxidants, and other nutrients vital to your health. The fiber and protein found in nuts also contributes to blood sugar regulation and fat loss. They also maintain hormone levels in your body that aid in burning fat, and are also a good food to keep your appetite lower and therefore reduce your general calorie intake. You can eat a handful of almonds, pecans, or walnuts up to a half hour before each meal to decrease your appetite and give you protein, fiber, and healthy fats. Raw nuts are better than roasted nuts, since the roasting process decreases the amount of healthy components in the nuts. Aside from whole nuts, you can also find a variety of nut butters that you can swap out from your ordinary peanut butter. Almond butter, pecan butter, and macadamia butter are good and tasty alternatives to add some diversity and nutrition into your diet.

Berries are a tasty way to add a whole bunch of vitamins and minerals to your diet, and also are one of the most antioxidant-rich foods there are. Berries also slow down carbohydrate absorption and digestion as a result of the fiber they contain, and also regulate blood sugar levels to avoid sudden increases in insulin.

Another healthy food that may surprise you is that of red meat. Although you hear often that red meat should be limited, this is simply because the majority of red meat that is easily available in the store comes from cattle that are fed an improper diet. Red meat found in grocery stores generally come from animals that are fed a diet consisting of grains, corn, and soy, which is not what they are naturally intended to eat. This disrupts the makeup and health of the animal, and thus produces meat of the same quality. A poor, unnatural diet can cause digestive issues within cattle that can result in e-coli, which warrants the use for antibiotics for the animal, which then become present in the meat it produces. Cattle that are fed an all-natural diet of grass and greenery produce meat that is considerably lower in omega-6 fatty acids and much higher in omega-3 fatty acids compared to their counterparts which are fed an unnatural diet. In addition, grass-fed cattle tend to have a much higher level of conjugated linoleic acid (another healthy fatty acid) and up to three times the amount of Vitamin E than grain-fed cattle. Conjugated linoleic acid has been shown to contribute to muscle-building and fat-burning. Grass-fed meat is a little more difficult to come by than grain-fed meat, but you can ask the butcher at your grocery store or find a specialty butcher that has organic cuts of beef.

LIVING HEALTHY WITH DIABETES

The main objective for anyone with diabetes is to have a low body fat percentage, which can be accomplished with a clean diet and consistent physical activity. The results can be major, even resulting in diabetes reversal. Aside from that, if you maintain this healthy lifestyle, you can steer clear from other diseases and have an overall longer, healthier, and happier life. In addition to keeping up a healthy diet and exercise regimen, it is also essential that you are aware of all of the lifestyle risk factors associated with diabetes and further complications, including smoking, stress, and sleep deprivation. Diabetes, if handled incorrectly, can take years off of a person's life, as well as make the lasting years less enjoyable with pain and discomfort. Although it is possible to reverse certain levels of diabetes, there is always a risk of it returning if the person relapses into an unhealthy lifestyle.

Below are a few lists of what people with certain levels and types of diabetes can expect from taking on a healthy, diabetes-friendly lifestyle:

PREDIABETES:

- No more spikes or severe decreases in blood sugar
- No more need for insulin
- No more need for diabetic medications
- Normal and maintainable body weight
- Longer, disease-free lifespan
- Less risk of complications from diabetes
- Overall increase in health

- More energy and endurance
- Complete eradication of diabetes

TYPE 2-DIABETES:

- No more spikes or severe decreases in blood sugar
- No more need for insulin within one week
- Need for diabetic medications reduced by half within the first week
- Decreased or discontinued need for diabetic medication within a month
- Normal and maintainable body weight
- Longer, disease-free lifespan
- Reversal of diabetes and less risk of complications
- Overall increase in health
- More energy and endurance
- Complete eradication of diabetes

TYPE 1-DIABETES:

- No more spikes or severe decreases in blood sugar
- Need for diabetic medications reduced by at least 50%
- Normal and maintainable body weight
- Longer lifespan with less risk of complications
- More energy and endurance
- If you have a relatively functioning pancreas, diabetes reversal and recovery of the pancreas and possibility to eliminate need for insulin
- Overall increase in health

KEEPING YOUR KITCHEN DIABETES-FRIENDLY

It is vital to make sure you have a healthy kitchen, free of high-carb foods and foods with fast-acting carbohydrates and sugars. Stock up on diabetes-friendly foods that you have read about in previous chapters. If you have housemates that don't follow this healthy lifestyle, store your food items separately from theirs, and label them so that no one takes them. It also helps to post a list of foods that you should avoid somewhere visible in your kitchen so that people you live with are aware. Also don't be afraid to ask your housemates for support and reminders if they ever find you slipping or deviating away from your healthy diet and lifestyle.

STAYING PHYSICALLY ACTIVE

Nothing can replace the need to maintain a healthy exercise regimen. It is known that people who exercise on a regular basis have lower insulin levels and are more sensitive to insulin. Diabetes has become more and more prevalent in our society lately due to the population becoming decreasingly active and thus overweight. Keeping active is especially beneficial to those with the most prevalent diabetic and heart disease risk factors. Exercise can reduce or even eliminate the need for diabetic medications, as it naturally lowers blood sugar levels. Lack of exercise actually ages the human body more than any other factor. You get tired more easily and more often, muscles weaken and lose mass, bones become fragile, skin becomes loose, posture becomes poorer, joints become more painful, and excess fat and weight put extra strain on your body to carry it. All of these things can at a certain point become life-threatening, resulting in chronic fatigue and making your body more susceptible to injury and illnesses. It is important, however, to realize that proper exercise varies from person to person. Many exercises can be beneficial to one person, while they can actually exacerbate the problems of someone else. Also, if you really feel the need to eat something with sugar or carbs, the best time to do it is immediately after exercising, since this is when your blood sugar is at its lowest level and glucose has been burned off. It is best to have a diverse exercise regimen, but the fact is that any exercise is better than none. You can even do something so small as to take the stairs instead of the elevator at work, or go for a walk during your lunch break instead of sitting down at a table or your desk.

It is best to do some kind of exercise every day, if possible in the morning. The human body was designed to be physically active on a daily basis, and when it is, metabolism is dramatically increased and calories burn off at a much higher rate. Weight training is one of the best forms of exercise you can do for both short- and long-term health benefits. It is important to space it out over the course of a few days (once every three days for a young person and once every four to five days for someone older) to allow for muscle rehabilitation following a workout. If you don't allow your muscles to rest and recover, it can actually have an adverse effect on them. The more toned and built up your muscles are, the more calories you will burn literally constantly, even while you are sleeping. Aerobic training also has many benefits, but with this kind of exercise the calorie burning is only consistent through the exercise itself and doesn't continue afterwards. Aerobic exercise also isn't aimed towards muscle building, but is still a great form of exercise. You can do aerobic exercise doing normal daily activities, such as parking farther away from the store while shopping so you can walk farther, or using the stairs instead of the elevator. There are a variety of different methods of aerobic exercise, including walking, biking, and swimming.

Walking at least a half hour every day is one of the easiest ways to incorporate exercise into your daily routine, seeing as it can be done throughout your day while you are doing other things. Another great alternative is biking. Biking is also very easy on the joints as opposed to running or jogging, and is a good form of aerobic and cardiovascular exercise. Because you are using the largest muscles in your legs, biking can actually burn the most calories of any other exercise, except that of cross-country skiing. You can get even greater results if you combine biking with doing sprints and interval training. You can also use a stationary bicycle to achieve the same results, but the nice part about using a regular one is that you can get out in the fresh air and view the scenery, making it less boring. There are also social groups and clubs that you can join with other like-minded individuals so that you can bike together. Because biking burns so many calories, if done regularly, you can be a little less strict with your diet. Using a bike outside is also free with no membership needed, which is even better. Besides doing it in your free time, you could try to incorporate biking into your daily commute, whether the entire way or part of the way if you must travel a farther distance. You can even ride a bike to the store and carry a backpack with you or attach another carrying bag or basket to your bike to bring back your purchased items. Swimming is also one of the best forms of exercise since it uses every muscle group in your body. There are a variety of different strokes you can try that focus on different muscles, while also adding variety to your workout.

Physical activity is an indispensable factor to facilitate weight loss and improve your health. If you remain regularly physically active, you can avoid and even reverse diabetes. The poorer of a physical state that your body is in, the more physical effort it will require. It is normal that if you are new to exercising, your endurance will be much lower in the beginning. This can be built up over time with slowly increasing the intensity of your workouts. Start off with numerous short periods of exercise per day, and eventually you will be able to withstand longer and more intense workouts. Although low-intensity workouts and cardio activities such as walking, jogging, swimming, and biking are beneficial to your body, nothing is more crucial than weight training and muscle building. Everyone begins to lose muscle mass at a rate of 0.5-1% per year beginning in the twenties. This increases weight gain as it decreases metabolism, since muscle burns the most calories in the body. There are two specific forms of exercise that are the most ideal for increasing muscle mass and your overall health, which will be explained in the upcoming sections. These two exercises are known as rebounding and slow-motion weight training.

REBOUNDING

Rebounding is one of the best forms of exercise you can do for your body, and on top of that, it's also fun! Rebounding is simply jumping up and down on a mini trampoline. It is even more quick and effective for weight loss than power walking, jogging, and swimming. It encourage weight loss through burning more calories, which is the main goal of many diabetics. It burns eleven times more calories than walking, five times more calories than swimming, and three times more calories than running. It can be a life-altering exercise for people with a variety of diseases, especially diabetes.

While rebounding, the immune system goes into hyper drive, tripling the activity of the white blood cells, which lasts for about an hour. White blood cells are the main defense mechanism that fights against disease and sickness. With their increased activity, they become busy eradicating cancer and other diseased cells, damaging microbes, and hazardous toxins. Even after just two minutes of rebounding, the spike in white blood cell activity lasts for an hour and then lowers back to normal. You can do short periods of rebounding through the day (ideally once an hour) to keep your white blood cell activity elevated to clean out harmful contaminants in your body and strengthen your immune system.

Unlike any other form of exercise, rebounding actually flushes your lymphatic system and enhances your immune system. The lymphatic system is your body's main method of decontaminating and cleansing your body and has a huge influence on the immune system, helping to prevent cancer, heart disease, and a variety of other serious health complications. The lymphatic system carries nearly four times the amount of fluid as compared to blood, and aids in proper digestion, heart function, auto-immunity (which is a problem in people with Type 1-diabetes), inhibits infections spreading, encourages protein balance, is anti-inflammatory, and more. Just two minutes of low-intensity rebounding can completely cleanse the entire lymphatic system, while also reinforcing and refreshing your cells. Since your lymphatic system is operated by gravity rather than by a pump (unlike the cardiovascular system), rebounding forces it into motion. Physical activity is therefore essential to cleanse the lymph nodes and lymphatic system, which is why many sedentary people tend to have lymphatic issues.

The best way to get the most positive effects out of rebounding is to do it for two minutes at a time at least once an hour. Doing small, low-intensity sessions throughout the day is actually more beneficial than doing one longer session. The effects are phenomenal, putting your immune system into action, empowering your cells providing them with more oxygen, and unceasingly flushing out your lymphatic system. Rebounding uses and strengthens all 638 muscles in your body, and when done regularly, it can also reduce or prevent cancerous tumors and improve or eradicate many other health conditions, including osteoporosis. Another great thing about rebounding is that you can do it anywhere at home, also while watching television or listening to music. If you have problems keeping balance, you can also purchase a stabilizer bar at the same place that you can buy your rebounder. If you don't want to purchase a stabilizer bar, it also helps to hold onto a vertical pole or even the back of a chair in your home for balance. After a short while, your balance will improve so that you no longer need additional support. You can start off slowly with shorter sessions and gradually increase to two-minute-long sessions, eventually repeating this numerous times throughout the day.

The positive effects of rebounding are enormous. In addition the flushing the lymphatic system and strengthening the immune system, it also counteracts fatigue and tiredness through enhancing the glandular system. This entails boosted activity in the thyroid, pituitary, and adrenal glands, creating an analgesic effect that releases chronic pain in the joints, neck, back, and head with improved oxygen and blood flow. This also results in the heart rate dropping, putting less stress on your heart and increasing circulation power. Rebounding is a great exercise for people who are less mobile or going through physical rehabilitation. For diabetics it is especially beneficial, as it decreases cholesterol and triglyceride levels, as well as heightens metabolism which leads to more calorie burning and weight loss. Endorphins are also released during rebounding, which make you feel good mentally as well as physically, as they act as a natural painkiller mood lifter. It can also slow down physical aging by keeping the heart and circulatory system healthily functioning. Digestion is improved, you get more sleep and relaxation, regulates nerve impulses, and mends muscle fiber. Nerve damage is a common effect of diabetes, so this is another reason why this is a good exercise for diabetics. It burns more calories than running or jogging and doesn't put the added stress on your joints, which is important to recover a diabetic body.

Rebounding is both fun and phenomenally valuable, providing countless health benefits throughout the entire body. There is no other exercise you can do that will cover so many physical issues. You can invest in a low-cost rebounder and do it in the comfort of your own home instead of paying money to go to a gym, and you get more bang for your buck.

SLOW-MOTION WEIGHT TRAINING

An increase in strength is best achieved through weight training, but high-intensity weight train is more likely to cause injury. There is an alternative, however, which is called "slow-motion" weight training. Instead of doing quick, long sets of repetitions, you work your muscle to its limit through smaller sets of very slow and drawn-out motions. Instead of rapid up-and-down movements, take your time with the lifting and letting down, spanning each separate movement over about ten seconds. Do a single set of four to six repetitions, and then you're done!

Slow motion weight training not only gives you great results, but also saves you a lot of time and added strain. You build up even more muscle mass than with regular strength training, increasing your calorie-burning rate dramatically, including when you are resting. Similar to rebounding, it also strengthens your bones, preventing and repairing bone damage and conditions such as osteoporosis, without the need for drugs or supplements. Bone density and muscle mass naturally decrease with age, generally beginning around the age of 25 at about 0.5%-1% per year. For women this is especially dangerous, since they are also more susceptible to osteoporosis. Through strength training, your circulation improves, your blood sugar levels regulate, and your body responds better to insulin that recover your blood pressure, cholesterol, and triglyceride levels. Upon achieving this, if you have diabetes you can gradually discontinue the use of drugs with negative side-effects, or even wipe diabetes off the table completely. Compared to the higher-intensity normal method of weight training, slow-motion weight training is done with a much lower momentum and does not forcibly fight against gravity at such a vigorous rate. You can thus greatly reduce your chances of muscle, ligament, tendon, and joint injury or damage.

Slow-motion weight training is ideal for elderly and younger people, putting less stress on the body and able to be done at home within a much shorter period of time. As opposed to normal strength training that achieve the same results in up to three hours, slow-motion weight training sessions can be completed in as little as 30 minutes. Also, with slow-motion strength training, all of your muscle fibers are put into use, whereas with conventional strength training only four muscle types are engaged. What's more is that slow-motion weight training combines cardio with strength training. It is unnecessary to do high-intensity, quick-motioned workouts that put added strain on the joints, ligaments, tendons, and bones when you can achieve even better results while at the same time saving your body from a lot of stress.

High-impact fitness activities such as jogging and some other cardio sports are much more likely to cause long-term damage to the joints and connective tissues. Many joggers and runners tend to develop chronic problems in as little as three years of regularly running. This doesn't mean that you need to give up sports that you enjoy like tennis, basketball, or others; it is important, however, that you remain aware of the risks with activities such as golf with quick, high-impact movements to avoid future complications with your body. Through strength training, your metabolism and muscle mass are exponentially increased, burning more calories both while active and at rest, whereas with cardio exercise, the fat-burning ceases immediately upon finishing the activity. Conversely, slow-motion weight training contributes to general fitness, increased muscle mass, weight loss, a long-lasting increase in calorie burning, improvement in bone density, and a much lowered chance of bodily injury and damage. Along with all of these benefits, it can be done in a vastly shorter amount of time than cardio or conventional strength training, and can save money on a gym membership with the purchase of some weights that you can use at home (or you could even use household objects in place of weights or dumbbells). So save your body time and strain by keeping off the treadmill or track and improving your body composition with slow-motion strength training!

REINFORCING THE IMMUNE SYSTEM

The key to a healthy and prolonged life, is a strong immune system. People often neglected the importance of a strong immune system and are often ignorant to their ability to strengthen and reinforce their immune system. The majority of your immune system, 60% to 80%, is situated in your stomach in the form of healthy bacteria. Simply put, it is not healthy for your stomach to have an abundance of bad bacteria, or to lack the good bacteria. The weaker your immune system is, the more susceptible you will be to a wide variety of sicknesses, such as the common cold, the flu, diabetes or even diseases as deadly as cancer and heart disease.

To better understand your immune system, it is important to understand all of its functions and all that it does for your body. There are two primary ways of which your immune system functions to keep your body healthy: Cell Mediated Immune Response and Humoral Immune Response. The two responses work in precise and detailed ways to prevent disease and sickness. Cell Mediated Immune Response functions by using specific cells that are an active part of your immune system and utilizing their actions. These specific cells include your T-lymphocytes (T Cells), which are a form of white blood cells that kill off dangerous pathogens such as viruses, fungi, harmful bacteria, and tumor antigens. These cells trigger your body's fighting cells that attack tumors, viruses and macrophages, which are essentially bigger cells that are able to attack and fight against disease-causing organisms. Another specific cell type that is a part of your immune system are Cytokines. Cytokines are proteins that activate your body's fighting cells, such as macrophages. Essential to the healing and repairing of wounds, Cytokines are able to quash all sorts of inflammations in your body. The second primary way of which your immune system keeps you healthy, is Humoral Immunity. It uses your antibody and antigen reaction to dangerous antigens and any harmful intruders. Special proteins known as antibodies, are formed by your body to help fight antigens and intruders including viruses, bacteria and toxins. Upon detecting invader antigens, your body's antibodies will destroy those invading antigens by attacking and sticking to their surface. Stress is a large contributor to your immune system's overall strength and healthy. This includes any kind of stress, such as emotional, financial, physical, and dietary stresses. When your body is stressed, it can weaken your immune system, leading to sicknesses and illnesses of all kinds. Your body's natural way of protecting you, is not something to be ignored or neglected. It isn't solely for the hopes of avoiding a common cold or flu, there is a much larger picture, that of which your entire life depends on the ability of your immune system to kill and attack deathly diseases as severe as cancer or heart disease, and even long term deadly diseases like diabetes. Research has provided us with countless ways to effectively improve your immune system, making sure it is in pristine condition. One proven way of doing so is probiotics and prebiotics. Recent studies have proven both to have the ability to enhance both Cell Mediated and

Humoral Immune Response, and stimulate the cells in your immune system. Throughout this text you will find countless more ways to effectively strengthen your immune system, enhance the quality of the life you live, and furthermore, prolong your longevity past your expectations.

Quality of life in this text, is defined as your life's vivacity, significant decrease in the frequency and length of sickness, and life prolongation, all due to a strong immune system's ability to fight against deadly, disabling and life-threatening diseases. An immune system suffering from diabetes is salvageable; simply consume one quart of Lifeway Kefir per day. If you wish to reinforce your already strong immune system, consume two quarts of Lifeway Kefir each week. To locate a source within close proximity, check out the Lifeway Kefir Website: http://lifewaykefir.com. Lifeway makes fermented liquid yogurts, similar to a smoothie, that are available in a variety of flavors. They contain protein for muscle and cellular growth, and they have added 12 beneficial probiotic bacteria that aid in the strengthening of your immune system and the improvement of your body's digestion. For more information, check out and read the labeling on the bottle – it's quite impressive. The problem with antibiotics, is that in addition to killing off the bad bacteria, they kill the good bacteria that makes up 60% to 80% of your immune system, which is your body's defense against disease. Lifeway Kefir offers probiotics, which is able to repair and restore your immune system. If you are interested, Lifeway Kefir will be located in the refrigerated dairy section, next to the coconut water.

An important step to take in better your immune system, is switching your meats, dairy products, and eggs to organic sources, including free-roaming animals that aren't fed Antibiotics, Steroids, or Hormones, and have a natural diet. The majority of the meat and dairy we consume, comes from animals that were given loads of antibiotics to keep them from getting sick. In order to steer clear of these types of products, read the label on the package, to ensure that your meats, daily products, and eggs do not come from sources that were raised with antibiotics in their systems. Mother Nature is Always Best: A favorite meat of mine is the wild Mahi and wild Alaskan Salmon. A private farmer supplies me with eggs from free-roaming chickens, raised on natural non-GMO feed that doesn't contain Antibiotics, Steroids, or Hormones. Try a natural alternative to sugar, such as Stevia. Sugars encourage the bad bacteria in our immune systems, allowing for bugs such as MRSA, other diseases like cancer and heart disease, and ailments such as diabetes. It's better to opt for the liquid form of Stevia, rather than powdered, as an anti-caching ingredient is often found in powders that are cut with a sugar-like dextrose. A few drops is all you need when it comes to Stevia, as it is naturally 400 times sweeter than sugar. My favorite Stevia brand is Now Foods, and you can find it on Amazon.com.

When picking a Stevia brand, read the label to ensure its 100%; some deceitful sellers will attempt to trick you, by adding only a little bit of Stevia into a sugar compound like dextrose. If you read the ingredients list and come across anything ending in "ose", it is a sugar (dextrose, fructose, sucrose, etc.). This deceitful substance is more often in powdered form. In addition to sugar, avoid sweet sugar-like substances such as molasses, honey, malt, agave nectar, and even some sweet fruits. Use caloric free Stevia as opposed to those artificial sweeteners if you wish to strengthen your immune system; they are also seen to increase weight gain. Jack LaLanne put in simpler words: "If man made it don't eat it don't put it on your skin". Stay clear of canola oils and switch to natural oils such as coconut. Another important thing to note, is to avoid fried foods unless you have done the frying yourself, in a natural oil such as coconut oil.

The Dangers of Antibiotic Overuse

Anyone who has taken antibiotics at any point most likely has a candida yeast growth in their body. This growth is usually found within the intestine, but there is a chance that it may spread throughout the body. This growth may cause a plethora of problems, including but not limited to common complaints such as headaches, heartburn, allergies, constipation, and nausea. In some occasions, it may even be a cause for more serious concerns, such as arthritis, diabetes, depression, or even fibromyalgia. One of the typical problematic side effects of a candida infection is the difficulty, or even incapability to lose weight. This can be problematic, as excess weight can lead to greater health problems, especially for diabetics. Excess candida growth causes food cravings, and signals the body to eat even when it doesn't need to. The removal of the candida can cause someone to lose weight without even trying, as their appetite will be reduced, usually to a normal level, cutting excess calorie consumption.

Another common use of synthetic antibiotics is through creams, lotions, and even antibacterial soap. These are commonly used topical products that disturb the balance of bacteria on the skin. Human skin produces its own natural antibiotic proteins, and overuse of these synthetic antibiotics may harm this balance.

The human body is designed to combat harmful infections on its own, through natural antibiotics. Everyone has live bacteria located in their intestines that aid digestion and help maintain a body's health. These bacteria also assist the body in fighting off harmful bacteria, but when someone takes antibiotics, both helpful and harmful bacteria are killed, ruining the body's balance. An example of this would be the use of antibiotic creams, lotions, and antibacterial soap on our skin. Our skin creates proteins that combat harmful bacteria, and the overuse of such products may damage the body's natural ability to fight off harmful bacteria. One way to avoid this is refraining from taking antibiotics unless absolutely necessary, and instead working on improving our body's immune system. A way to do this is to employ the use of supplements such as vitamin C, Zinc, and prebiotics and probiotics, all of which help bolster the body's immune system. These supplements aid the body in the following manner: Vitamin C assists the immune system through stimulating the body's manufacture of white blood cells, which fight off infections. Echinacea is an herb that keeps the body's lymphatic system healthy as well as helps purify the blood. Zinc is a mineral used by the body to develop stronger resistances against infections. Garlic is one of the best antibiotics that is readily available to us, as it helps in killing bacteria as well as building the immune system, to the point that garlic may be able to help treat minor infections of the ear, mouth, and throat. Carob powder is a supplement that helps the body deal with diarrhea. Aloe vera is an antiseptic and an antibacterial that helps treat sore throats, disinfect the skin, and even helps in the restoration of injured tissues. Grapefruit seed extract is a supplement commonly used to help treat skin rashes, as well as bacterial strains like staph, salmonella, and strep. Honey is an antibiotic that is effective on minor skin injuries such as bites and cuts, and is often used to treat asthma. It can totally prevent the growth of harmful bacteria. Colloidal silver hinders the growth of certain strains of bacteria, and is used to treat damaged tissue both inside and outside the body. However, care needs to be exercised when using colloidal silver as overuse may lead to a buildup in the body, causing grey skin. The oil of the tea tree is an antiseptic used to treat fungal infections, yeast infections, and halitosis. Molkosan and Olive leaf extract are some supplements that aid in the treatment of fungal and yeast infections. Olive leaf extract has also been reported to help in the regulation of blood glucose levels, as well as the treatment of high blood pressure. Bitter melon is another fruit often used to lower blood sugar levels, and may be used to treat infections in the gastrointestinal tract. Slippery elm is used to treat respiratory problems such as excessive mucous, bronchitis, and bleeding in the respiratory system. Neem is a plant that has antiseptic, antiviral, and antipyretic characteristics, and is also often used as a blood purifier. These are just some examples of natural supplements that we can use to improve our immune system to reduce the need for synthetic antibiotics. Overuse of synthetic antibiotics can lead to the development of antibiotic-resistant bacteria, as well as the unbalancing of the body's natural bacteria.

Maintaining the Right Attitudes and Beliefs

Many factors are involved in our well-being and success, but one of the most important ones is our state of mind. One of the biggest reasons of failure is the lack of belief in one's own capability to succeed. A significant contributor to this poor mental outlook is the simple lack of the knowledge needed to achieve one's goal. Someone who is equipped with the proper knowledge and the correct attitude will be able fully motivated and will be able to commit their complete dedication towards the completion of their goals. A person's mental attitude can make or break their progress towards their goal. People who believe in themselves will keep trying, and will not be discouraged by failure, as they will see it as a temporary setback. Someone who has a negative attitude, however, will absolutely fail, since they will not try to begin with. A person's mental attitude affects not only themselves, but their environment as well. People who are upbeat and optimistic tend to attract people of a similar disposition, creating an environment of support, allowing them to more easily reach their goals. People who are negative and pessimistic, on the other hand, will attract people similar to them as well, creating a negative environment that further hampers or even halts their progress towards their goals.

A person who wants to change their attitude can begin by changing their environment. By culling the negative factors in a person's life, they can begin to change. Getting rid of toxic people and replacing them with those that are genuinely supportive will also be a big factor in changing a person's mental attitude.

Mind over matter is real, and one example of this would be the placebo effect. The placebo effect is a well-known phenomenon wherein someone that believes that something will help him actually gets helped by it, even though there is no real basis for it, other than their own belief. For example, in many double blind studies, around a fifth of the subjects who take the placebo will show signs of improvement, due to their belief that taking the pill will help them. This is a testament to the power of belief and positive thinking.

Good health does not mean mere physical wellness. Good health, when taken holistically, includes a person's mental and spiritual health, as well as their attitude towards life. Though a person can be in good physical condition, if their attitude is negative, their condition may worsen. Conversely, someone who is afflicted with a disease can improve their recovery by maintaining a positive attitude.

This is due to certain changes that affect the body due to a person's mental attitude. For example, someone who produces too many stress hormones will weaken their own immune system, rendering them more vulnerable to diseases. More often than not, a person's mental health directly affects their physical health.

One of the ways to maintain a positive attitude is by taking life as it comes. As the saying goes, when life gives you lemons, make lemonade. Looking at the bright side of things will help immensely in lowering stress levels and in maintaining a positive outlook. Something that also greatly helps in maintaining positivity is a person's belief system. No one's belief system is necessary better or more valid than another's, as it is a matter of personal choice. Each person's beliefs should be given the proper amount of respect. Believing in something, however, allows someone to maintain a sense of stability and balance in their life.

One more method of maintaining positivity is creating something similar to a "Vision Board". A vision board is a method wherein pictures and images of a person's goals is attached to a board, and placed somewhere that it well be seen frequently. These pictures and images do not necessarily have to be of material things, but they may be of any type of goal one has. Beside each image, the date when the goal should be completed is placed. In addition, the steps to achieve the goal should also be written down. This process helps in visualizing the achievement of the goal, and creates encouragement and positive reinforcement towards it.

The Dangers of Diabetes

Diabetes is caused by the malfunction of the pancreas. The pancreas is a unique organ that performs both endocrine and exocrine functions. Most of the pancreas' cells work on the digestive side, known as the exocrine side, while about 5% is composed of endocrine cells, known as islets of Langerhans. It is a 6 inch long gland that lies within the abdomen, between the stomach and the spine. It connects to the small intestine, through the duodenum. It produces hormones that help in digestion and the body's regulation. Some of the primary hormones produced by the pancreas include insulin and glucagon, which help regulate blood glucose. Insulin regulates glucose by allowing the body's cells to absorb and use glucose. Glucagon works in reverse, stimulating the body's cells to release glucose and raising blood glucose levels. Somatostatin is another type of pancreatic hormone that is secreted by the pancreas that maintains the balance of glucose and salt in the body. The pancreas also produces gastrin, a hormone that aids digestion, by inducing the stomach to produce acid. Another important hormone is vasoactive intestinal peptide, a hormone that controls water emission and absorption from the intestine by inducing intestinal cells to release water and salts into the intestines. Without a proper balance in hormones, the human body is prone to serious disorders, such as diabetes. There are two types of diabetes, Type 1 and Type 2. Type 1 diabetics don't produce enough insulin for their body to use glucose properly, so they need constant insulin supplements. Type 2 diabetics are able to produce insulin, but their bodies aren't able to use it correctly.

Diabetes in all forms, including prediabetes, is a condition that increases the likelihood of developing long-term complications. It typically develops over many years, and is often left undiagnosed. Diabetes increases the mortality rate of affected individuals, regardless of other factors such as age, sex, or race. The leading cause of death of those affected by diabetes is heart disease. The primary complication of diabetes is damage to small blood vessels, including damage to the eyes, kidneys, and nerves. Diabetes doubles the risk of heart disease, with up to 60% of diabetics dying as a result of coronary artery disease. Other common causes of death are strokes, which account for almost 25% of deaths in diabetic patients, as well as peripheral vascular disease.

A possible complication of diabetes is a low blood glucose crisis, also known as hypoglycemia, or insulin shock. This occurs when blood sugar levels drop below 70 mg/dl. Low blood sugar counts are common in people with type 1 and type 2 diabetes who use insulin supplementation and drugs. Hypoglycemia may also be caused by inadequate ingestion of food, overproduction of glucagon, excess exertion, or intake of alcohol. Most cases, however, are mild and not considered medical emergencies. Mild cases of hypoglycemia is most often found among type 2 diabetics, and serious episodes are uncommon, even for those who are taking insulin. All diabetics should be knowledgeable of the symptoms, however, especially those taking diabetic medications. When hypoglycemia occurs, effects may include feelings of unease, abnormal sweating, trembling, weakness, rapid heartbeat, and increased hunger. Mild cases may be easily self-treated through ingesting food or drink with a high level of sugar. In certain cases, hypoglycemia abruptly appears, and if left unattended, may easily escalate. A recent prior episode of hypoglycemia may make it more difficult to detect when it reoccurs. This may be avoided through vigilant monitoring and avoiding low blood glucose levels. However, even careful monitoring may fail to detect a problem, especially if it occurs during sleep. Hypoglycemia may become severe or even life threatening, especially when a patient fails to be aware of their symptoms, and continues taking insulin supplements or other drugs that cause hypoglycemia. Severe cases may lead to the loss of consciousness, and is treated through intravenous glucose or glucagon injections. If left untreated, severe hypoglycemia may lead to confusion, behavioral changes, infections, or even permanent brain damage or death. In certain cases, hypoglycemia appears suddenly, and if left unattended, may easily escalate.

Diabetic patients, especially those with type 1 diabetes, may also experience episodes of diabetic ketoacidosis. Diabetic Ketoacidosis, or DKA, is a life threatening disorder caused by insulin deficiency. Until recently, it was most often found in type 1 diabetics who were noncompliant with their insulin supplementation. However, cases of Diabetic Ketoacidosis have been increasingly reported in those with type 2 diabetes as well. It is not definitively known what causes the depletion of the hormone insulin in these patients. Signs of diabetic ketoacidosis include excess thirst, high blood sugar level (hyperglycemia), fruity-scented breath, and confusion. These symptoms may develop quickly, sometimes even within 24 hours. If left unattended, DKA may lead to a metabolic disturbance characterized by nausea, vomiting, excessive urination, abdominal pain, the smell of acetone on the breath, deep breathing known as Kussmaul breathing, and in severe cases a decreased level of consciousness or coma, or even death. DKA may be detected through home blood and urine ketone testing kit. Anyone with diabetes who feels ill or stressed, or who has undergone a recent illness or injury should check their blood glucose level often. If a diabetic begins to vomit and cannot tolerate food or liquid intake, or their blood glucose level begins to increase to levels over the target range, they should immediately contact their doctor, as it is possible that they may have an elevated ketone level.

Hyperosmolar Nonketotic State, or HNS, is a dangerous form of diabetic coma. This comatose state is also known by other terms such as hyperosmolar hyperglycemic nonketotic coma, or hypersomotic non-ketoic acidosis. This complication often arises in diabetics. This condition is caused by the rise of blood sugar levels, and the human body tries to cleanse the excess blood sugar by creating more urine. If abnormal feelings of thirst persist despite increased liquid intake, it is possible that a person has HNS. If sufficient liquids are not imbibed, the body may become dehydrated, leading to the development of HNS, often lasting several days or months. A diabetic must watch out for signs and symptoms of HNS, as if left unattended, it may lead to major complications. Some symptoms of HNS include the body having a blood sugar level over 600 mg/dl that does not drop over time, continuous feelings of unquenchable thirst, dry skin due to a lack of sweating, a parched mouth, fever, weakness affecting one side of the body, or even confusion, hallucinations, blurred vision, and sleeplessness.

Cardiovascular disease and diabetes are closely linked, and diabetics often develop cardiovascular diseases early on, often even before their diabetes is diagnosed. There is a high association between high blood pressure, or hypertension, unhealthy cholesterol levels, and diabetes. Medical studies suggest that high LDL ("bad" cholesterol), low HDL ("good" cholesterol), as well as high triglyceride levels, all interfere with insulin regulation. The Standard American Diet, or SAD, has created a nation wherein up to 86% of the population is considered overweight or even obese. The Standard American Diet is a diet with low nutrients, high carbohydrates, low protein, and bad fats, leading to high rates of heart disease, cancer, diabetes, and many other diseases. The low micronutrient food of the standard American diet provides inadequate nutrition, and encourages consumption of excess calories, leading to the high incidence of obesity. Hypertension is more often found in diabetics versus non-diabetics. Diabetes affects the cardiovascular system in numerous ways, such as speeding the progression of atherosclerosis and having low HDL and high levels of triglycerides. This may lead to coronary artery disease, a heart attack, or a stroke. Diabetes may also cause impaired nerve function, or neuropathy, causing heart abnormalities. Women with diabetes are at an even more elevated risk level for heart problems and death from heart disease.

Atherosclerosis is a condition wherein the arteries in the body begin to harden, often caused by a high-calorie diet. Excess consumption of calories leads to a buildup of plaque and cholesterol in the arteries. Food low in macronutrients, such as processed food, increases oxidative stress through the creation of free radicals, and inflammation, which accelerates the development of arteriosclerosis. Both types of diabetes have also been found to accelerate the progression of atherosclerosis. Another cause of inflammation is thought to be through showering in chlorinated municipal water, as the chlorine is diffused by the showerhead and is inhaled, leading to scarring of the lungs and arteries.

Neuropathy is one of the most common complications of diabetes, being a group of disorders that affects the nervous system. It is an early side effect of diabetes that is caused by elevated blood sugar levels. Even "mildly" raised blood glucose levels barely above 140 mg/dl may case neuropathy, and up to half of type 2 diabetics have detectable neuropathy at the time of diagnosis. It is also possible to never be diagnosed with diabetes and yet be afflicted with diabetic neuropathy. Diabetic neuropathy is a major cause of impotence among men in their 40s and older. Signs of neuropathy often begin in the feet, with a tingling or burning sensation. There are two major types of neuropathy autonomic neuropathy and peripheral neuropathy. Peripheral neuropathy affects nerves in the limbs, affecting the toes, feet, legs, hand, and arms. This type of neuropathy affects sensation, and is a complication that affects almost half of the diabetics who have been afflicted for 25 years or more. Peripheral neuropathy's symptoms generally begin in the extremities, and move up the arms and legs. These symptoms include itching, burning sensations, weakness, and the loss of sense of warm or cold. Autonomic neuropathy affects the nerves that aid in the regulation of digestive, bowel, bladder, and sexual functions. This condition may cause digestive problems such as constipation, diarrhea, nausea, and vomiting. It may also cause bladder infections, incontinence, erectile dysfunction, or even heart problems.

Nerves affected by neuropathy will eventually lose sensation. After a doctor has diagnosed a patient with diabetes, they should test the patient to check for dead nerves. This test is carried out on a patient's feet using a tuning fork or a thin filament in order to check for the presence of dead nerves that the patient may not have noticed. If a doctor does not check for neuropathy after diagnosing you with diabetes, consider looking for a different doctor. This is because neuropathy is a very common ailment afflicting diabetics, and the occurrence of neuropathy in a patient's feet suggests that other nerves in the body are under attack. One of the nerves that get damaged by an elevated blood sugar level is the vagus nerve, a nerve that serves as the link between the brain and the rest of the body, and serves to regulate the immune system. This is why diabetics often have trouble fighting infections, as a damaged vagus nerve hampers the immune response. The nerves in the extremities may also die if neuropathy is left unattended. Simply treating the symptoms, but ignoring the underlying cause may lead to irreparable damage. Neuropathy causes nerves to fail because the blood vessels that supply the nerve become clogged. This stops the ability of the body to send white blood cells to fight the infection of the affected tissues. This leads to gangrene and possible amputation.

The pain caused by neuropathy may mask angina, the warning sign of heart disease or an impending heart attack. Patients with diabetes should be aware of warning signs of a heart attack, including sudden fatigue, sweating, shortness of breath, and nausea and vomiting. The progress of neuropathy may be halted and even reversed, however, with tight control of blood glucose levels, lowering triglycerides, losing weight, reducing blood pressure, and quitting smoking. Strict control of blood sugar levels is highly encouraged, and one way to do this is by following a diet tailored for diabetic patients.

Another side effect of diabetes is kidney damage. Kidney damage may result in the scarring of certain tissues, protein loss through urine, and even chronic kidney disease, or CKD, requiring dialysis or a kidney transplant. Chronic or permanent kidney failure may occur in 20% to 40% of diabetes patients. One factor that may lead to kidney failure is high blood pressure. An elevated blood pressure level leads to large protein molecules, especially those that are glycosylated (enclosed with excess glucose), being pushed through the pores of the kidney's filtration units, leading to kidney damage. Another factor leading to kidney failure is a high level of blood sugar. When the body's glucose regulation fails, the kidneys remove excess glucose from the blood, leading to a high concentration of glucose in the kidney. The glucose clogs up capillaries in the kidneys, damaging and destroying the glomeruli, the kidney's filtration units. When glomeruli are damaged, they leak proteins into the urine. This eventually leads to kidney failure. This can be detected through testing for the presence of microalbuminuria (presence of protein) in the urine. Symptoms of kidney failure include inflammation in the lower extremities, itching, exhaustion, and a pale skin color.

Another possible effect of diabetes is damage to the eyes. This is called diabetic retinopathy. Retinopathy means "sick retina", and this is one of the scariest complications of diabetes. It is caused by damage to the blood vessels that supply the retina. This results in the gradual loss of vision and may lead to total blindness. The longer a person has diabetes, the higher the likelihood of developing diabetic retinopathy. Diabetes causes the annual development of thousands of new cases of blindness, and is the leading cause of blindness in adults age 20 to 74. Diabetes sufferers also have an elevated risk for developing cataracts as well as certain types of glaucoma, such as a condition known as primary open angle glaucoma, or POAG. The risk for POAG is especially high for women affected with type 2 diabetes.

Retinopathy usually occurs in two phases: the more frequent type of retinopathy is called non proliferative or background retinopathy. The blood vessels in the retina are weakened, and may rupture and leak, forming waxy areas. Once these affect the central portion of the retina, swelling may occur, causing reduced or blurred vision. If capillaries become blocked and cut off blood flow, soft, "woolly" areas may form in the retina's nerve layer. These woolly areas signal the development of proliferative retinopathy. This is a more serious condition wherein new atypical blood vessels form on the retina's surface. These may spread into the eye cavity or bleed into the back of the eye. Major hemorrhage or retinal detachment may result, causing loss of vision or even blindness. One sign of this is having the sensation of seeing flashing lights, indicating possible retinal detachment. When the eye is continuously exposed to high blood sugars, the small blood vessels located in the retina begin to grow in a uncontrollable and haphazard fashion. These diabetic blood vessels have weak walls, leading them to eventually burst, and releasing blood into the eye. If this is untreated, these blood vessels will ultimately destroy the retina's capability to convey images to the brain, resulting in permanent loss of sight. Prolonged elevated blood sugar levels may cause glucose absorption in the lens of the eye, which leads to shape changes, resulting in vision changes, cataract formation, or blindness. Another type of diabetic retinopathy is called macular edema, which refers to inflammation in the portion of the retina that grants central vision. Diabetes drugs such as Actos and Avandia have been discovered to lead to a possible increase in the cases of macular edema, causing doctors to recommend not taking these drugs if possible. The treatment of retinopathy is the use of lasers to close bleeding blood vessels in the eye. This stops the degradation of vision, but it does not restore lost vision. However, if blood sugar levels continue to be elevated, especially when at a level of 200 mg/dl or more, deterioration may continue regardless of treatment. The way to stop diabetic retinopathy is to lower blood sugar levels to normal levels to stop the damage. Blood sugar should be maintained at a normal level, not just a level considered "good for diabetics", in order to totally avoid the effects of retinopathy.

Patients who suffer diabetes are much more prone to develop problems with their tendons. This is because by nature, the supply of blood to the body's tendons is already sparse, so changes in the body's blood vessels due to diabetes tend to affect the tendons first. Another reason is that high blood sugar levels may cause the abnormal thickening of the body's tendons. Typical forms of damage common to diabetics and prediabetics are carpal tunnel syndrome, tarsal tendon syndrome (a form of carpal tunnel syndrome that affects the feet), and frozen shoulder. Around 15% of diabetics have are afflicted with severe foot problems. These are among the leading causes of hospitalizations for these patients. In fact, diabetes is the cause for more than half of all lower limb amputations performed in the US. There are about 88,000 non-injury amputations performed in the US each year, and diabetes accounts for 50-75% of these operations. About 85% of these amputations begin through foot ulcers, which affect around 12% of diabetic patients. Those who have the highest risk level are long-time diabetics or diabetics who are obese or overweight or are smokers. Those who are at the highest risk are diabetics who have had the disease for more than 20 years, and are insulin dependent. Other risk conditions are peripheral neuropathy, peripheral artery disease, foot deformities, and ulcers. Foot ulcers tend to develop from infections, such as those that result from blood vessel injuries. Even though it may start as a minor condition, these may eventually develop into more serious complications. This is compounded by the fact that numbness due to damage to the nerves, common in diabetics, may lead a patient to be unaware of their injuries.

One type of foot complication is called Charcot's foot. This is a foot disorder caused by congested blood vessels. This complication is caused by years of exposure to elevated blood sugar levels. In this condition, the long bones of the foot are deprived of nutrients due to damage to the circulatory system, and break, causing the collapse of the foot. This condition is crippling and may lead to gangrene, as the damage to the body's circulatory system prevents the immune system from transporting white blood cells to the affected area. This condition, also called neuropathic arthropathy, has been found to occur in up to 2.5% of diabetics. Early signs appear similar to an infection, with the foot beginning to swell, becoming red, and becoming abnormally warm. Gradually, the foot becomes deformed, leading the bones to crack, splinter, and erode. The joints may shift, change shape, and become unstable as well. This is often found in people who have neuropathy, as they cannot feel sensation in their feet and are thus unaware when there is an injury. Charcot's foot is treated with the strict immobilization of the foot and ankle; oftentimes, a cast is used. After the initial danger has passed, patients are usually given a brace and custom footwear to use for the rest of their lives.

Diabetes may also cause a series of rashes, blemishes and sores, and these are known as diabetic dermatomes. Diabetics are at increased risk for bacterial infection of all kinds, especially on the skin. This type of infection is even more serious for those who do not properly control their diabetes, such as those do not follow a diabetic diet. Infection with staph bacteria, or its treatment-resistant mutations, known as the Superbug MRSA is especially dangerous. This may cause sores, styes, boils, folliculitis, and even deep infections. There is also an increased risk for fungal infections that may affect the nails, genital area, and feet. Body folds may darken and thicken due to insulin resistance. This condition is called acanthosis nigricans, an early symptom of diabetes. Diabetic dermopathy is another condition wherein injuries to small blood vessels in the skin cause brown spots on the legs. Granuloma annulare presents as spherical or arc-shaped lesions due to changes in the skin's collagen. This condition has been linked with diabetes, especially when the condition becomes widespread.

Diabetes may also affect the brain's cognitive function. Studies indicate that patients with type 2 diabetes face an elevated risk level of dementia caused by Alzheimer's disease or blood vessel problems in the brain. Problems in attention and memory may occur even in people under the age of 55, especially when they have suffered diabetes for a number of years. Diabetics are also at a heightened risk for depression, being twice as likely to develop depression. This may increase the risk of hyperglycemia and other complications of diabetes.

Respiratory infections are also more common in diabetics, with diabetics facing a higher risk for influenza and its complications, including pneumonia, due to diabetes neutralizing the effects of the protective proteins in the lungs. Diabetes also leads to an increased level of risk for other disorders, such as periodontal disease, carpal tunnel syndrome, nonalcoholic fatty liver disease, also known as nonalcoholic steatohepatitis (NASH), especially for those who are considered obese or overweight. It may also increase the risk of certain types of cancer, such as colorectal cancer and uterine cancer.

Certain complications of diabetes are unique to women. Certain types of medications, such as birth control pills, may raise blood glucose levels. The long term use of these pills may increase the risk of health complications. Thiazolidinediones, a type of diabetic medication, may prompt ovulation in premenstrual women, and may reduce the effectivity of birth control pills. Diabetes may also decrease vaginal lubrication, leading to pain or discomfort during sexual intercourse. Women with diabetes are also at a notably elevated risk for UTIs, or urinary tract infections, which also tend to be more complicated and difficult to treat. Both gestational diabetes, (a type of diabetes only occurring during pregnancy) and pre-existing diabetes may increase the risk for birth defects. Studies indicated that an elevated blood sugar level may affect the developing fetus, especially during the first 6 weeks of organ development. It is therefore important for women with diabetes who plan to become pregnant maintain proper glucose control for a few months before pregnancy, and maintain it until delivery. The shift in estrogen levels as well as in other hormones that transpires during perimenopause may also affect blood glucose levels. Women with diabetes may also face an increased risk of premature menopause, leading to a greater risk of heart disease.

Diabetes also has complications specific to men. Unexplained muscle mass loss may be a taken as a warning of elevated blood glucose levels or even diabetes. If blood sugar levels remain elevated for long periods during the day, the body begins to break down fat and muscle for energy. This causes rapid weight loss, and is usually the most noticeable in people with type 1 diabetes. However, it may also affect people with type 2 diabetes, especially if left undiagnosed for a long period of time. Men who are affected with diabetes may also be afflicted by erectile dysfunction. This is caused by an elevated blood sugar level causing problems with the penis' blood supply, as well as possibly causing injuries to nerves located in the penis. Men may also be afflicted with a condition called genital thrush. This is a yeast infection that may occur due to high blood sugar levels, causing excess sugar to be flushed out by the body through urine. This causes redness, swelling, and itching around the head of the penis, as well as producing an unpleasant odor.

The Right Doctor for You

When traditional medical practices fail a patient, it may be wise to seek out practitioners of alternative medicine. There are doctors who practice naturopathic and integrative holistic medicine that may be able to help where traditional medicine fails. These doctors' treatments incorporate nature, certain types of alternative medicine, and scientific research. They often go above and beyond the Hippocratic oath to "do no harm".

These doctors prefer to treat the disease rather than prescribing artificial medicines to combat the diseases' symptoms. They may be difficult to find, but certain doctors are well-known, such as Dr. Andreas Grossgold. There may even be a naturopathic doctor near the area, as one may easily be found by searching online.